Social Indicators Research Series

Volume 57

This new series aims to provide a public forum for single treatises and collections of papers on social indicators research that are too long to be published in our journal *Social Indicators Research.* Like the journal, the book series deals with statistical assessments of the quality of life from a broad perspective, It welcomes the research on a wide variety of substantive areas, including health, crime, housing, education, family life, leisure activities, transportation, mobility, economics, work, religion and environmental issues. These areas of research will focus on the impact of key issues such as health on the overall quality of life and vice versa. An international review board, consisting of Ruut Veenhoven, Joachim Vogel, Ed Diener, Torbjorn Moum, Mirjam A.G. Sprangers and Wolfgang Glatzer, will ensure the high quality of the series as a whole.

More information about this series at http://www.springer.com/series/6548

Filomena Maggino
Editor

A New Research Agenda for Improvements in Quality of Life

Springer

Editor
Filomena Maggino
Dipartimento di Statistica, Informatica,
Applicazioni "G. Parenti" (DiSIA)
Università degli Studi di Firenze
Firenze, Italy

ISSN 1387-6570 ISSN 2215-0099 (electronic)
Social Indicators Research Series
ISBN 978-3-319-15903-4 ISBN 978-3-319-15904-1 (eBook)
DOI 10.1007/978-3-319-15904-1

Library of Congress Control Number: 2015937192

Springer Cham Heidelberg New York Dordrecht London

Printed on acid-free paper

Springer International Publishing AG Switzerland is part of Springer Science+Business Media (www.springer.com)

A New Research Agenda for Improvements in Quality of Life

As known, quality-of-life studies have a long history and inherited the tradition of the "social indicators" movement, aimed at supporting public administrations and interested in gathering and analysing data aimed at studying non-economic components of societal wellbeing. Between ups and downs, quality-of-life issues and researches roused scholars' interest not only in the academic world.

In 1974, the scientific journal *Social Indicators Research, An International and Interdisciplinary Journal for Quality-of-Life Measurement* and during the 1990s *International Society for Quality-of-Life Studies* (ISQOLS – www.isqols.org) were founded and became reference points for the movement.

Starting from the 1990s, ISQOLS organized several international conferences around the world (Canada, USA, Spain, Germany, South Africa, Italy, and Thailand).

All ISQOLS conferences have been and are occasions for lively debates, involving statisticians, sociologists, psychologists, physicians, economists, architects, communicators, educators, civil servants, and other experts. This made the discussion transversal, captivating and engaging, leading to the developments of many networks, like the one involving community wellbeing studies.

This vitality aimed also at urging quality-of-life topic to be put in the policy agenda and among policy goals all around the world.

That is because one of the most important aims of those conferences is to verify if it is possible to move this important and essential aspect of wellbeing, quality of life, from the academic world's agenda also to policy's agenda.

In this perspective, it is particularly important that the ISQOLS network is able to improve the research agenda in the field of quality-of-life studies. This was particularly evident in the context of the XI ISQOLS conference.

Following the great success of the IX conference, which took place in 2009 (July, 19–23) in Florence, ISQOLS conference was back to Italy. In fact, the XI conference took place in another extraordinary Italian city, Venice, in November 2012. The event was organized with the organizational support of the Italian Association for Quality of Life Studies (www.aiquav.it).

In Venice, many contributions were able to outline a possible new research agenda for improvements in quality-of-life research. The new orientation includes identifying and studying subpopulations and subgroups, disentangling the difficult task of identifying determinants of quality of life, refining the capacity of measuring conceptual dimensions, defining new indicators able to measure and monitor particular social conditions and show that these are not separated fields of studies but intersect each other and produce different outcomes which can be with difficulty classifiable, consistent with the idea of the complexity of our reality.

This volume represents a (small, if we compare it to the many papers presented) collection of some of the most interesting papers presented in that occasion.

The articles illustrate micro perspectives by taking into account the macro situation through both qualitative and quantitative approaches.

Some of them deal with national projects, identifying particular and relevant domains of wellbeing (*Well-being indicators on landscape and cultural heritage: the experience of BES project*) or aiming at constructing comprehensive accounts of all the assets of a country in order to assess the sustainability of its development path (*Towards Satellite Accounts on Education and Human Capital in OECD Countries*).

A particular ambit of quality-of-life studies, always considered of great interest, is represented by the analyses of determinants. This kind of studies needs to be focused not only on general population perspective but also on subgroups (*Determinants of student satisfaction with campus residence life at a South African university* and *Explaining the Ethnic Minority Disadvantage in Subjective Well-being: A Multilevel Analysis of European Countries* and *Associated factors to leisure activities in Quality of Later Life*).

Quality-of-life studies have to explore different methodological perspectives in order to study new social phenomena (*Dimensions of quality of living: An ethnographic research in two neighbourhoods of social housing*), take into account the relationship between the individual and the community perspective (*Making the Extraordinary Ordinary: A Fresh Look on Individual Action with Communities*), and relate objective and subjective dimensions (*Self-evaluation Affects Subjective Well-being: The Effects of Socioeconomic Status and Personality on Quality of Life in Taiwan* and *The Impact of Public Expenditures on Chinese Elders' Life Satisfaction* and *The Incidence of the Need for Personal Assistance and Care: Objective Living Conditions and Subjective Assessments*).

We believe that this volume represents not only a good evidence and proof of what was presented at the XI ISQOLS conference but also an inspiring collection of topics. This collective work, showing contributions by young and "less young" researchers, testify how this research field is not only lively in the present but also promising for the future.

Last, but not least, I would like to thank the anonymous reviewers of the papers, who made a great work and assured a high scientific quality of the publication.

Filomena Maggino
Chair of XI ISQOLS conference

Contents

Chapter 1
Well-Being Indicators on Landscape and Cultural Heritage: The Experience of the BES Project

Luigi Costanzo and Alessandra Ferrara

The BES Project

The BES project (where BES stands for *Benessere Equo e Sostenibile* – "equitable and sustainable well-being") was launched in Italy in 2011, on a joint initiative of Istat and CNEL,[1] in the wake of the international debate on "going beyond the GDP". The project is aimed at "measuring and assessing the progress of Italian society" by putting in place, within the framework of official statistics, the regular production of a set of well-being indicators. The BES project largely builds on the results of the *Commission on the Measurement of Economic Performance and Social Progress* (henceforth the Stiglitz Commission), convened by the French government in 2008, whose final report was published in September 2009.[2] To implement the project, a Scientific commission was established at the end of 2011, open to representatives of a wide range of civil society organisations, and a first report on "equitable and sustainable well-being in Italy" was published in March 2013.[3]

The idea underlying the project is that the GDP is improperly being used far beyond its original scope, relying on the assumption that the well-being of a population is a linear function of its market production of goods and services. For a number of reasons, after the World War II the GDP became the main benchmark for policy making worldwide, despite Kuznets himself – who first proposed this

[1] Istat (*Istituto Nazionale di Statistica*) is the National statistical office of Italy (www.istat.it), CNEL (*Consiglio Nazionale dell'Economia e del Lavoro*) is the advisory body of the Italian Government and Parliament in matters of economy and labour market (www.cnel.it).

[2] Stiglitz et al. (2009).

[3] Istat and CNEL (2013). To know more about the BES project, see www.misuredelbenessere.it

L. Costanzo (✉) • A. Ferrara
Social and Environmental Statistics Department, Istat, Rome, Italy
e-mail: lucostan@istat.it; ferrara@istat.it

F. Maggino (ed.), *A New Research Agenda for Improvements in Quality of Life*,
Social Indicators Research Series 57, DOI 10.1007/978-3-319-15904-1_1

aggregate in 1934 – had warned against its use as a measure of welfare.[4] The adequacy of indicators of economic performance based on GDP figures, however, is being questioned since a long time, and substantial concerns have been raised mostly about their relevance as measures of social well-being, since the aspects of social and environmental sustainability of the economic growth are not taken into account.[5] In brief, the project's challenge is to measure the performance of the society as a whole, conceived as something wider and more complex than the performance of its economy, in order to propose – both to policy makers and citizens – an alternative and more comprehensive view of progress and growth. This led to adopt the multi-dimensional approach recommended by the Stiglitz Commission, according to which the current macro-economic indicators should be complemented – not replaced – by indicators that reflect the people's quality of life, including measures of the inequalities and divides that undermine social cohesion, as well as measures of economic, social and environmental sustainability: "the time is ripe (. . .) to shift emphasis from measuring economic production to measuring people's well-being. (. . .) Changing emphasis does not mean dismissing GDP and production measures. (. . .) This means working towards the development of a statistical system that complements measures of market activity by measures centred on people's well-being and by measures that capture sustainability".[6] The implications of such a shifting are potentially enormous: to choose what official statistics shall measure, monitor, and bring to public attention is to define the priorities of economic policy; and to implement statistical information systems so conceived and oriented may significantly contribute to a deep cultural change, because "what we measure affects what we do".[7]

As a first step, the Coordination committee, a steering group composed by experts of both Institutions, defined 12 domains, each identifying a specific *dimension* of well-being. Of these, eight match (although not exactly) those proposed by the Stiglitz Commission (see Table 1.1). The four additional ones were introduced as a result of an extensive consultation process, carried out in order to get, as far as possible, to a widely shared vision of what people deem relevant to well-being, also in relation to possible singularities of the Italian case.

This way of proceeding was essential to the project's strategy, which is based on a participatory approach. The responses given to a specific question addressed to 24,000 households within a sample survey,[8] the results of a special web survey conducted among the users of the project's website (answered by 2,500 people), the

---

[4] Kuznets (1934), p. 7 ("The welfare of a nation can scarcely be inferred from a measure of national income").

[5] See Costanza et al. (2009, 2014). For a comprehensive review of the various approaches to the measurement of individual well-being and social welfare that have been considered for the construction of alternatives to GDP (and for an extensive bibliography on this subject as well), see Fleurbaey (2009).

[6] Stiglitz et al. (2009), p. 12.

[7] *Ibidem*, p. 7.

[8] The Istat survey on *Aspects of daily life*, carried out on a yearly basis (edition 2011).

Table 1.1 Well-being dimensions proposed by the BES project and by the Stiglitz Commission

BES project	Stiglitz Commission
Health	Health
Education and training	Education
Work and life balance	Personal activities including work
Economic well-being	Material living standards (income, consumptions and wealth)
Social relationships	Social connections and relationships
Politics and institutions	Political voice and governance
Safety[a]	Insecurity, of an economic as well as physical nature[a]
Subjective well-being	
Landscape and cultural heritage	
Environment	Environment (present and future conditions)
Research and innovations	
Quality of services	

[a]The BES dimension of *Safety* does not include the "insecurity of an economic nature", which falls under *Economic well-being*

discussion – both on the project's blog and in several public meetings – of a number of spontaneous contributions received from experts in various disciplines, were all part of a complex decision process. Eventually, the Scientific commission was tasked with implementing a subset of relevant indicators for each dimension and, after a new debating phase, released a list of 132 indicators, on which basis the first BES Report was finally compiled (a chart of the decision making process is provided in Fig. 1.1).[9]

In synthesis, the Report is meant to provide every year an overview of the Italian society, focused on the qualitative aspects of its development and seeking to evaluate the current trends in terms of their effects on people's well-being. In each of the 12 dimensions identified, a positive evaluation is given to those dynamics that appear to be *equitable* (i.e. likely to enhance or at least not to reduce the social cohesion) and *sustainable* in the long term (i.e. not based on consumption of non-renewable resources, and not imposing burdens on the future generations). To take into account the well-known inequalities that characterise the Italian economy under the territorial profile, it was planned to produce each indicator both at the national and at the regional level,[10] also in order to provide a useful benchmark instrument for regional policies.

[9] Documentation of the BES Project in English is available at http://www.misuredelbenessere.it/index.php?id=documents

[10] The 21 NUTS 2 units (19 Regions and 2 autonomous Provinces), according to the current EU classification of territorial units for statistics, set by the Regulation (EC) No. 1059/2003 and subsequent amendments.

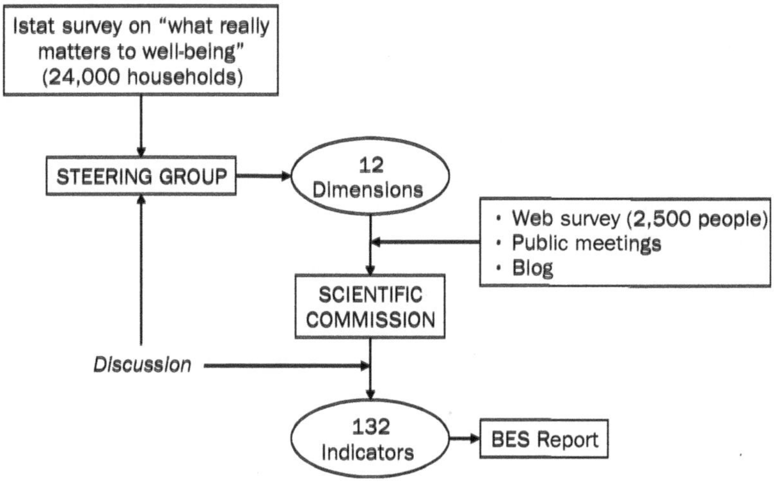

Fig. 1.1 Development of the BES project

Landscape and Cultural Heritage as Well-Being Factors

This article focuses on one of the dimensions proposed by the BES project in addition to those identified by the Stiglitz Commission – *Landscape and Cultural Heritage*, which are considered under their aspect of *common goods* of a non-renewable nature, whose preservation is deemed relevant to well-being.[11] The decision to devote to this topic a dimension of its own was made after nearly 80 % of respondents of the above mentioned web survey had indicated this as one of the dimensions "most relevant" to well-being. Famously, Italy boasts an

[11] In the sense that is generally accepted in the economic theory, *common goods* are defined as goods that are *rivalrous* (because their consumption by one person precludes consumption by another one) and *non-excludable* (because no payment is required in order to use them), whereas *public* goods are non-rivalrous and non-excludable. Here, we refer to the more inclusive definition proposed by the Rodotà Commission, established by the Italian Ministry of justice in 2007 in order to modify the Civil code regulations in matter of public goods, according to which goods shall be distinct into private, public and common, and the latter are defined as "things that express utilities functional to the exercise of fundamental rights and to the free development of the individual. Common goods must be protected and safeguarded by the legal system, also for the benefit of future generations. Holders of common goods can be either public or private legal persons. In any case, it must be ensured that these goods are available for collective enjoyment, to the extent and in the manner established by the law". This applies, in particular, to "the river streams and their sources, lakes and other waters; the air; the parks, as defined by law, the forests and woodlands; the mountain areas of high altitude, glaciers and permanent snows; the beaches and coastlines declared environmental reserves; the protected wildlife and flora; the sites and properties of archaeological, cultural and environmental interest, and any other protected landscape areas" (Ministero della giustizia 2007). The reform bill proposed by the Rodotà Commission was presented to the Senate, but never came to parliamentary debate.

extraordinary cultural heritage, both in quality and quantity. The management of this immense wealth, however, suffers from insufficient funding, while the Italian landscape is being threatened by one of the highest illegal building rates over Europe. Maybe to a wider extent than in other countries, the issues linked to heritage and landscape conservation assume, in Italy, a special relevance in relation to some crucial aspects of the societal performance, such as the care for public assets and the management of conflicts between private and public interest. In this regard, it is worth remarking how the Italian Constitution (1948) mentions the protection of "the landscape and the historic and artistic heritage of the Nation" among its "fundamental principles",[12] while "landscape and cultural heritage" are the joint subject of the Code that has unified and renewed the whole Italian legislation on the matter in 2004.[13]

Initially, it was needed to set up a conceptual framework for the domain to be investigated, which was largely new to quantitative analysis. It was deemed useful to start from the classic distinction proposed by the Italian geographer Biasutti (1962) between "geographic landscape" (an abstract image, synthesising the most recurring or significant elements that characterise the visible form of a territory) and "sensible landscape" (the subject of individual perception).[14] On one hand, the *sensible landscape* pertains to the *subjective* sphere, and can be considered relevant to individual well-being – insofar the landscape of daily life has an influence on the people's quality of life, depending on a variety of factors (not only of an aesthetic nature but also emotional, symbolic, etc.). The *geographic landscape*, on the other hand, pertains to the *objective* sphere, and can be considered relevant to collective well-being – insofar it provides any significant witness of the local history, tradition, or material culture. A landscape that has been shaped into specific forms along the course of history confers a special identity on a given part of the territory, and on this identity (or, more exactly, on the shared acknowledgement of it) relies the cultural value of a landscape, and its status of common good (heritage) to be preserved.

A first assumption we can make, then, is that the geographic landscape can be regarded as an integral part of the cultural heritage, being the result of a long interaction between mankind and nature (see Fig. 1.2). This does apply, however, only to *urban* and *rural* landscapes, and does not to *natural* landscapes, whose value relies on their environmental qualities, and primarily in the absence or insignificance of any form of anthropic alteration – which is just the opposite of what makes a landscape valuable from the cultural point of view. Therefore, with

---

[12] *Costituzione della Repubblica Italiana*, art. 9. For a critical history of the Italian legislation on landscape protection, see Settis (2010).

[13] *Codice dei beni culturali e del paesaggio* (Legislative Decree no. 42 of 22nd January 2004).

[14] Biasutti (1962) defines the *sensible* (or *visible*) landscape as "what the eye can embrace, or (...) is perceptible to all senses; a landscape that can be reproduced by a photograph (...), the work of a painter or the description of a writer", while the *geographic* landscape is defined as "an abstract synthesis of the visible landscapes, which tends to detect the elements or features that present the most common repetitions over a given space (...), which is larger, in any case, than any space encompassed by a single horizon".

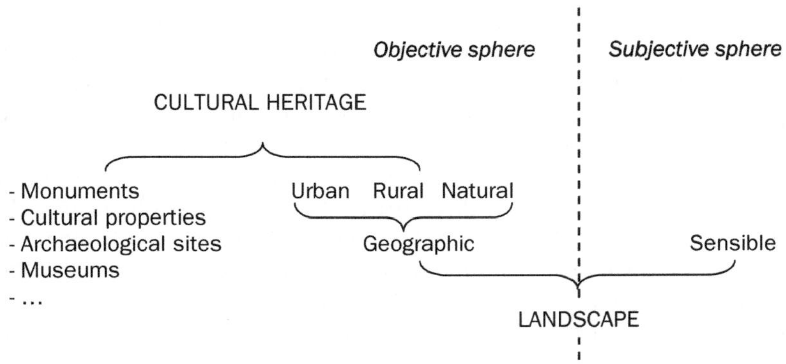

Fig. 1.2 Conceptual framework

regard to the objective sphere, only urban and rural landscapes are considered relevant to this domain, while, within the BES framework, the natural landscapes pertain to the Environment dimension, insofar their contribution to collective well-being essentially coincides with that deriving from the conservation of protected areas such as national parks, natural reserves, etc.[15]

With regard to the subjective sphere, instead, the landscape is considered in its entirety, as a general concept, without distinction between natural, urban and rural areas, and solely as an object of individual perception. In this case, what we consider relevant is the landscape of the places we live in (home and neighbourhood, working places, commuting trips, etc.), while the occasional enjoyment of other landscapes as travellers or tourists should be rather considered as a form of cultural consumption, like visiting an exhibition or going to the cinema – experiences that also contribute to individual well-being, but in another way and to a different extent.

Basically, the sensible landscape, being the subject of individual perceptions, can be investigated only by means of a survey, and synthesised as the sentiment of respondents in relation to the landscape of the places where they live. To this goal, a couple of experimental items were included in the questionnaire of the Istat sample survey on "Aspects of Daily Life", starting from 2012. It is possible, instead, to obtain measures relating to the cultural heritage (including the geographic landscape), although mostly of an indirect nature, based on existing data sources of various nature.

A set of well-being indicators on landscape and cultural heritage should therefore contain both measures referred to *subjective aspects* – to evaluate the

[15] Measures of the conservation of protected areas were developed within the Environment dimension of BES. See, in particular, the indicators *Terrestrial parks* (Ratio of the surface of terrestrial protected areas to the total surface), *Marine protected areas* (Extension of marine protected areas) and *Areas of special naturalistic interest* (Ratio of the surface of areas belonging to the EU network "Natura 2000" for the conservation of biodiversity to the total surface).

contribution (positive, negative or null) of the sensible landscape to the quality of life of individuals, and measures referred to *objective aspects* – to evaluate the state of the cultural heritage as a common good, of which the present and future generations have the equal right to enjoy.

Indicators Proposed for the Subjective Aspects (Sensible Landscape)

The indicators proposed to capture the subjective aspects of this dimension of well-being derive from two questions purposely included in the Istat survey on "Aspects of Daily Life": (1) *Do you consider the landscape of the place where you live affected by evident degradation?* [*Yes/No*], and (2) *Which of the following environmental issues are you most concerned about? (5 responses allowed)* [*Greenhouse gas, ozone hole/Extinction of animal/vegetal species/Climate change, global warming/Waste production and disposal/Noise/Air pollution/Soil pollution/Pollution of seas and inland waters/Events such as earthquakes, floods, landslides, etc./ Deforestation/Electromagnetic pollution/Decay of landscape due to overbuilding/ Exhaustion of natural resources/Other (to be specified)*].[16] The first question is meant to detect situations of extreme hardship, which are associated – in the perception of interviewees – to a negative characterisation of the landscape as the setting of daily life; while the latter aims to measure – against other environmental issues – the social concern about the protection of the landscape. Through these questions it is sought to capture two key aspects of the landscape as the object of individual experience – the need for a pleasing landscape as a factor of life quality, and the awareness of the landscape's value as a common good. The proposed indicators are:

- *People that are not satisfied with the quality of the landscape of the place where they live* – Proportion of regional population reporting that the landscape of the place where they live is affected by "evident degradation". In 2012, the overall share of unsatisfied people was 18.3 %, but this figure highly varies by region along the North-south axis (from 6.8 % of Trento Province to 31.1 % of Campania), largely echoing the general economic conditions of the individual regions.[17]
- *Concern about landscape degradation* – Proportion of regional population reporting, among the "most concerning" environmental problems, the "decay of landscape due to overbuilding". People who mentioned this among the five "most worrying environmental issues" were 20.4 % of the total in 2012, against 15.8 % of

[16] The first question has been introduced in 2012, while the second had been already used in 1998. From 2012 onwards, both questions will be submitted every year. For the time being, it was preferred not to overload the questionnaire (quite demanding already) with further questions on this topic.

[17] Source: Istat, *Aspetti della vita quotidiana* (2012).

1998. Figures significantly vary according to education levels (from 17.7 % among lower education levels to 26.7 % among the higher ones – the same gap recorded in 1998, witnessing a persistent social divide in the sensitivity to environmental issues). Also in this case, however, the greatest variability can be observed at the territorial level. The concern is more felt, and increased more, in the North (from 18.5 % of 1998 to 25.3 %), less so in the Centre (from 14.4 % to 18.9 %) and even less so in the South (from 13.0 to 14.6 %).[18]

Indicators Proposed for the Objective Aspects (Cultural Heritage, Including the Geographic Landscape)

To analyse the geographic landscape, it was proposed a partition of the territory in three main "phases" (urban, rural, natural), each characterised by specific problems and different evaluation parameters, focusing on urban and rural landscapes, as parts of the cultural heritage. It was also agreed to give emphasis to some cross-cutting themes of a special relevance in Italy, such as the endowment of heritage items and the related expenditure by the local authorities for management and conservation, as well as the plague of illegal building.

Within the geographic landscape, special attention was paid to the component of *rural landscapes*, whose protection was one of the main objectives of the "National strategic plan for rural development" (2007–2013), where the landscape is regarded as "a fundamental resource resulting in a value added for the products with designation of origin, instrumental to the development of tourism as well as for the biodiversity of cultivated areas, and a key factor for life quality in rural areas".[19] In Italy, home to an ancient and pervasive anthropisation process, rural areas cover the far larger part of the territory, but also the more vulnerable one, as regards the landscape. While the protection of historical centres and natural areas is well settled in the regulatory framework and widely passed into common sense, the conservation of rural landscapes is still struggling to be recognised by legislation and, even more, to aggregate a broad consensus among the public opinion. The selection and industrialisation of the most profitable crops, the abandonment of traditional farming practices (mostly in mountain areas), the competition between farming and real estate in urban surroundings, are still largely perceived as acceptable (if not desirable) dynamics of modernisation and economic development, regardless of their collective costs – not only in terms of a loss of cultural and biological diversity, but also in terms of environmental degradation and hydro-geological instability. The current crisis of the rural space in Italy can be compared to an *erosion process*, acting on two fronts – urbanisation and re-naturalisation. In other words, as shown in Fig. 1.3, the residual stable or active farming areas are losing ground in favour of

[18] Source: Istat, *Aspetti della vita quotidiana* (1998 and 2012).

[19] Ministero delle politiche agricole, alimentari e forestali (2010), p. 26. See also: Ministero delle politiche agricole, alimentari e forestali (2007, 2009).

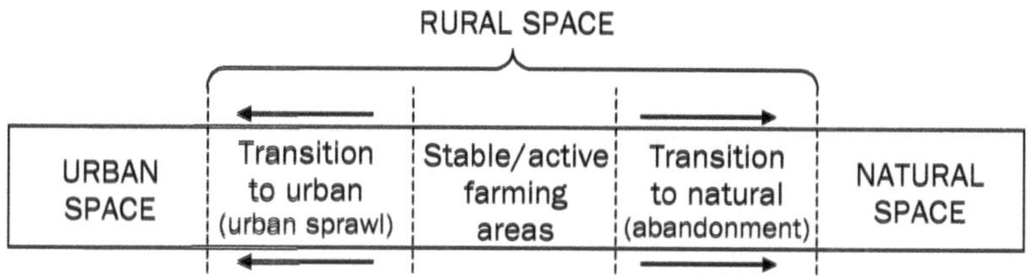

Fig. 1.3 Erosion of rural space

vast transition (erosion) areas, either invaded by the low-density urbanisation that stretches out from the outskirts of consolidated towns (so-called "urban sprawl") or abandoned by farmers and returning to some kind of wilderness.

Ten indicators, briefly presented below, have been developed in relation to the aspects of the cultural heritage and geographic landscape:

(Cross-cutting indicators)

- *Endowment of cultural heritage items* – The number of archaeological sites, monuments and museums surveyed by the "Risk Map of Cultural Heritage" (an information system held by the Ministry of Heritage and Cultural Activities), per km^2. This indicator allows representing a territorial distribution of the cultural heritage. At the end of 2012, there were more than 100,000 items surveyed across Italy (on average, 33.3 per 100 km^2). The regions where a higher density of heritage items combines with a relatively low population density (such as Umbria, Marche and Tuscany), appear to be in the best position to protect and valorise their patrimony as a factor of collective well-being, as well as to fully exploit its potential for territorial marketing.[20]
- *Expenditure of Local authorities for the management of cultural heritage* (museums, libraries and art galleries), per capita. In times of shrinking of public spending, and competition between public services for funding, an above average share of spending on culture is a good indicator of the sensitivity of local communities to cultural issues. Italian Municipalities provide about 45 % of the national public spending on culture – on average, € 10.5 per capita (2010). Regional mean values follow the territorial distribution of income, ranging from less than € 5 per capita in Southern Italy to € 12 in Central, up to € 14 in Northern Italy.[21]
- *Illegal building rate* – Ratio of the number of unauthorised buildings to the number of building permits issued by the Municipalities. This indicator points out a key aspect of governance – the protection of public goods against the private speculation. Illegal building not only harms the landscape, but undermines the credibility of local governments and encourages negative behaviours

[20] Source: Elaboration from Ministero per i beni e le attività culturali, *Carta del rischio del patrimonio culturale* (2012).

[21] Source: Elaboration from Istat, *Bilanci consuntivi delle amministrazioni comunali* (2010).

and expectations. Taking advantage from a wide social tolerance, this phenomenon has reached proportions that are uncommon in Europe: it equals approximately the 5 % of legal building production in the North, 10 % in the Centre and 30 % in the South – where a major upturn seems to have taken place in correspondence with the current economic crisis.[22]

- *Urbanisation rate of areas subject to building restrictions by virtue of the Italian laws on landscape protection* – Number of buildings realised after 1981 in areas subject to building restrictions by virtue of the Law no. 431/1985, per km^2. The so-called Galasso Law of 1985[23] imposed a general building restriction on coastlines, inland waters, mountain areas and other areas of a special environmental interest. A count of the buildings erected in these areas (legally or not) provides a direct measure of the pressure exerted on contexts of a special environmental value. In the coastal areas, the most attractive for building development, there were, on average, 437 buildings per km^2 in 1981. Twenty years later (after more than 15 years of enforcement of the Galasso Law) the figure rose up to 540 buildings per km^2 (+23.6 %).[24]

(Indicators relating to rural landscape):

- *Erosion of farmland from urban sprawl* and *Erosion of farmland from abandonment* – Ratios of the surface of agricultural districts affected respectively by urban sprawl (anomalous decrease of cultivated farmland + anomalous increase of extra-urban population[25]) or by abandonment (anomalous decrease of cultivated farmland + anomalous decrease of extra-urban population) to the total of the regional territory. This couple of indicators are calculated through a single classification procedure, applied to sub-regional observation units (the "agricultural districts").[26] Areas affected by urban sprawl cover 20 % of the national territory with generally higher values in the Centre-North, while the erosion from abandonment has an overall greater impact at a national level (28.3 %), but is less concentrated, with a slight prevalence in the South. Considering both forms of erosion, the provinces of Trento and Bolzano are the areas where rural spaces appear to be least threatened. The same applies, to a lesser extent, to

---

[22] Source: Cresme estimates on illegal building (2011) and Istat, *Statistiche sui permessi di costruire* (2011).

[23] Recast in the Legislative Decree no. 42 of 22nd January 2004 (*Codice dei beni culturali e del paesaggio*).

[24] Source: Elaboration from Ministero per i beni e le attività culturali, *Carta del rischio del patrimonio culturale* (2012) and Istat, *Censimento generale della popolazione e delle abitazioni* (1981 and 2001).

[25] Extra-urban population: people living outside the boundaries of the "inhabited localities", as surveyed by the Population Census.

[26] The agricultural districts (*regioni agrarie*) are territorially continuous clusters of Municipalities belonging to the same Province and class of altitude, and homogeneous by the market value of crops, which are established for Land registry purposes. Italy is divided into about 800 agricultural districts. The classification procedure is described in Costanzo and Ferrara (2013).

Piedmont, Tuscany, Umbria, Puglia, Sardinia, Friuli-Venezia Giulia and Marche, while the most critical situations appear to be those of Liguria and Veneto.[27] The transformation of large portions of the countryside into low-density suburbs, where often productive, commercial and residential uses mix with residual cultivated areas, is the outcome of a no longer sustainable development model, based on high soil consumption and increasing dependency from private mobility for commuting, with obvious negative consequences for both individual and collective well-being.

- *Presence of historical rural landscapes* – A score that takes into account the ranking of the Regions by the number and surface of the sites classified as such by the National inventory of historic rural landscapes (a project of the Ministry of Agriculture, Food and Forestry Policies, in progress).[28] If we consider the historical landscapes – especially where they are the outcome of traditional practices still in use – as an integral part of a local cultural heritage, this indicator can be seen as a necessary complement to the *endowment of cultural heritage items*.
- *Quality assessment of Regional programmes for rural development (PSRs), with regard to landscape protection* – Score assigned to the PSRs by a Commission convened by the Ministry of Agriculture, Food and Forestry Policies in 2009, based on an assessment of the potential impact on rural landscape of the measures adopted within the National strategic plan for rural development 2007–2013. The general objectives of agricultural policy set out by the EU and the national government (including the protection of rural landscapes) are implemented through planning instruments that are designed at the regional level. Although sharing a common framework, such instruments can greatly differ from a qualitative point of view, depending on the adequacy and feasibility of the envisaged measures. The PSRs deemed most likely to have a positive impact on the landscape are those of Umbria, Veneto, Valle d'Aosta e Friuli-Venezia Giulia.[29]

(Indicators relating to urban landscape):

- *Presence of historical parks/gardens and other urban parks recognized of significant public interest* – Parks and gardens classified as "historical" and/or "of a significant public interest" by the Legislative Decree no. 42/2004 in the provincial capitals (sq km per inhabitant). This indicator can be seen as another measure of *endowment*, referred to a specific component of the urban landscape. The overall surface of green areas and parks of historic or artistic interest that fall

[27] Source: Elaboration from Istat, *Censimento generale dell'agricoltura* (1990 and 2000) and *Censimento generale della popolazione e delle abitazioni* (1991 and 2001).

[28] Source: Elaboration from Agnoletti (2011).

[29] Source: Ministero per le politiche agricole, alimentari e forestali, *Paesaggio e sviluppo rurale. Il ruolo del paesaggio all'interno dei Programmi di Sviluppo Rurale 2007–2013* (2010).

under the protection of the Code of cultural assets and landscape covers about 5 % of urban areas.[30]

- *Conservation of historical urban centres* – Ratio of inhabited buildings realised before 1919 and in excellent or good state of conservation to the total number of inhabited buildings realized before 1919.[31] Like for the rural landscapes, the conservation of historical centres is relevant to well-being as long as these are vital and maintained in good conditions. Based on the latest available Census data (2001), almost two buildings in ten, on the total of inhabited buildings (2001), were built prior to 1919, 60 % of which are still in excellent or good state of conservation. In Tuscany and Umbria, such proportion rises to nearly 75 %, while it is below 50 % in Campania, Calabria and Sicily.[32]

A Critical Commentary on the Indicators Proposed and Some Concluding Remarks

Undoubtedly, the two indicators proposed for the subjective sphere (*People that are not satisfied with the quality of the landscape of the place where they live* and *Concern about landscape degradation*) can provide only a limited representation of the complexity underlying the relation between well-being and the perception of landscape, leaving unexplored – among other things – any influence that the town planning or the architecture of public spaces may have on subjective well-being. Moreover, the concern about landscape degradation is being measured only in relative terms, through a comparison with other environmental issues – which is likely to affect the comparability of data over time, insofar occasional emergencies may alter the respondents' rankings in the short term (not to mention any change in the response categories). The regularities found in the distributions of frequencies are consistent with well-known socioeconomic and territorial divides that characterise Italian society, proving that a structure exists in the relation between living conditions and the perception of landscape. On this basis, the subjective aspects of well-being relevant to this domain can be further developed within the framework of the BES Project, essentially by widening and consolidating the instruments for data collection. Currently, the landscape is represented only as a potential source of discomfort. Widening this representation so to consider also the benefits that may derive from the daily experience of a friendly and pleasant urban landscape, for instance, could lead to a more comprehensive view of the relation of people with the

[30] Source: Istat, *Dati ambientali nelle città* (2011) and *Basi territoriali dei Censimenti* (2010).

[31] The year 1919 was chosen as a plausible turning point between the prevalence of traditional building technologies and the diffusion of the technology of reinforced concrete.

[32] Source: Elaboration from Istat, *Censimento generale della popolazione e delle abitazioni* (2001).

places they live in. More generally, a clearer separation, on the survey questionnaires, of the conceptual domain of landscape (and cultural heritage) from that of environmental issues, could improve accuracy and relevance of the statistical measurement.

The indicators proposed for the objective sphere are mainly affected by problems of timeliness, because much of the data used come from the Censuses of Agriculture and Population, and are collected every 10 years. In addition, the validation process of some of the input data produced by these sources tends to be quite long: the 2011 Census data on population by enumeration districts, as well as those on buildings by year of construction, had not been released yet in 2013, which explains why the indicators of *erosion of the rural space* and that of *conservation of historical centres* refer to 2001. Also the *quality assessment of Regional programmes for rural development* cannot be updated every year, as its periodicity is clearly bound to the cycles of the EU and national agricultural policies. Different data quality issues regard the indicators of *endowment of cultural heritage items* and *presence of historical rural landscapes*, whose updating depends on the implementation of inventories that are managed for purposes other than statistical and, in the case of the *Catalogue of historical rural landscapes*, are still at an early stage of development. The enumeration of heritage items made by the *Carta del rischio*, on the other hand, is made on a regional basis, and the consistency of the inclusion criteria from one region to another, as well as the alignment of the updating operations, cannot be ensured. Nevertheless, these sources provide the best available basis for a quantitative measurement of heritage and historical rural landscapes in Italy.

Among the dimensions of well-being identified by the BES project, that of landscape and cultural heritage can be considered as one of the most pioneering ones, since it explores a field that is largely new to official statistics. Most weaknesses of this study can be linked to this exploratory approach, as well as to the tight schedule assigned to the Scientific commission to synthesise in a shared output a variety of inputs received from a wide range of interlocutors. In particular, the conceptual framework needs to be further developed and consolidated, also in order to organise the definitions and measures into a more homogeneous set. Crucial shortcomings have been identified as regards the available sources. In relation to landscape, in particular, which is essentially a dynamic entity, it would be most needed to develop a time series approach, but this is seriously limited, for the time being, by the poor usability of data from historic censuses, most of which are still not available in digital form, neither for the needed territorial detail. At the same time, the demand for relevant information related to this domain should be taken into account in the planning of future surveys, with special regard to the Censuses of population and agriculture – as well as it would be useful to collect more information on subjective perceptions and opinions on this matter: although of a clear evidence, the relationship between landscape, heritage and the quality of life has been only marginally considered so far in the domain of official statistics. A functional disaggregation of expenditure items within public administration balance sheets would be also needed, to make possible a more accurate identification of the resources actually allocated to cultural heritage management (presently melted into the generic container of "spending for culture").

The picture of the Italian situation composed by the proposed indicators – although greatly variable by Region – was correctly synthesised, in the first BES Report, as "a great wealth, not adequately protected" (Istat and CNEL 2013). The state of the heritage and landscape reflects the ability of a community to make good use of its own most valuable resources: recognising, preserving and valorising them as common goods. The extraordinary importance of Italy's cultural heritage appears to be largely underestimated in the allocation of public spending, while the landscape suffers from both the pressure of overbuilding and the radical changes in farming, that led since the 1960s to the abandonment of vast areas of the countryside – more generally, it can be said that a major issue is the poor attention paid by most local authorities to town planning and territorial governance. The resulting hardship is being increasingly felt by a not marginal share of the Italian population, in terms of dissatisfaction for the landscape of the place where they live and concern for the landscape degradation – which is a worrying sign for a country that, for centuries, has been named the "garden of Europe".

References

Agnoletti, M. (Ed.). (2011). *Paesaggi rurali storici. Per un catalogo nazionale*. Roma-Bari: Laterza.

Biasutti, R. (1962). *Il paesaggio terrestre*. Torino: Utet.

Costanza, R., & *alii*. (2014). Development: Time to leave GDP behind. *Nature, 505*, 283–285. http://www.nature.com/news/development-time-to-leave-gdp-behind-1.14499

Costanza, R., Hart, M., Posner, S., & Talberth, J. (2009). *Beyond GDP: The need for new measures of progress*. Boston: Boston University Press.

Costanzo, L., & Ferrara, A. (2013). *Misure statistiche per l'analisi del paesaggio rurale: l'esperienza del progetto BES*. Palermo: XXXIV Conferenza italiana di scienze regionali. http://www.grupposervizioambiente.it/aisre_sito/doc/papers/costanzo.doc

Fleurbaey, M. (2009). Beyond GDP: The quest for a measure of social welfare. *Journal of Economic Literature, 47*(4), 1029–1075. http://www.aeaweb.org/articles.php?doi=10.1257/jel.47.4.1029

Inter-institutional Initiative CNEL/Istat on the Measurement of Progress in Italy, Coordination Committee. (2011). *Proposal for domains*. http://www.misuredelbenessere.it/fileadmin/upload/docPdf/Cnel_Istat_committee_BES_domains.pdf

Istat, & CNEL. (2013). *BES 2013. Il benessere equo e sostenibile in Italia*. http://www.misuredelbenessere.it

Kuznets, S. (1934). *National income, 1929–1932*. 73rd US Congress, 2nd session, Senate document no. 124. http://library.bea.gov/u?/SOD,888

Ministero della giustizia. (2007). *Commissione Rodotà per la modifica delle norme del codice civile in materia di beni pubblici (14 giugno 2007). Relazione*. http://www.giustizia.it/giustizia/it/mg_1_12_1.wp?contentId=SPS47617

Ministero delle politiche agricole, alimentari e forestali. (2007). *Piano strategico nazionale per lo sviluppo rurale 2007–2013 (art. 11 Reg. Ce 1698/2005)*. Roma. http://www.reterurale.it/flex/cm/pages/ServeAttachment.php/L/IT/D/D.557b91d96fa77e0a96d5/P/BLOB%3AID%3D342

Ministero delle politiche agricole, alimentari e forestali. (2009). *Paesaggio e sviluppo rurale. Il ruolo del paesaggio all'interno dei Programmi di Sviluppo Rurale 2007–2013*. Roma. http://www.reterurale.it/flex/cm/pages/ServeAttachment.php/L/IT/D/D.557b91d96fa77e0a96d5/P/BLOB%3AID%3D342

Settis, S. (2010). *Paesaggio Costituzione Cemento*. Torino: Einaudi.

Stiglitz, J. E., Sen, A., & Fitoussi, J.-P. (2009). *Report by the Commission on the Measurement of Economic Performance and Social Progress*. www.stiglitz-sen-fitoussi.fr

Chapter 2
Determinants of Student Satisfaction with Campus Residence Life at a South African University

Ferdi Botha, Jen Snowball, Vivian de Klerk, and Sarah Radloff

Introduction

Campus-based student residences provide accommodation to many students every year as they pursue their academic studies. The quality of such accommodation and its environment are imperative in facilitating student learning and well-being. In a wider sense, the importance of residential characteristics in enhancing human well-being has been well documented. Rojo-Perez et al. (2001) and Prieto-Flores et al. (2011), for instance, have shown that residential satisfaction is an important predictor of elderly individuals' well-being, where being satisfied with the particular residence reduces negative emotions such as loneliness.

Despite the acknowledged importance of residence characteristics in fostering individual well-being, investigations into the predictors of student campus-based residence quality of life (QoL) are severely lacking. In South Africa, moreover, some reports have indicated certain campus-residence issues, though no study on South African universities has examined how factors experienced by students in residence are associated with their satisfaction with residence life. In general, research on QoL among South African university students is very scant. A study by Møller (1996) examined the dynamics of life satisfaction among University of

F. Botha (✉) • J. Snowball
Department of Economics and Economic History, Rhodes University, Grahamstown, South Africa
e-mail: f.botha@ru.ac.za; j.snowball@ru.ac.za

V. de Klerk
Division of Student Affairs, Rhodes University, Grahamstown, South Africa
e-mail: v.deklerk@ru.ac.za

S. Radloff
Department of Statistics, Rhodes University, Grahamstown, South Africa
e-mail: s.radloff@ru.ac.za

F. Maggino (ed.), *A New Research Agenda for Improvements in Quality of Life*, Social Indicators Research Series 57, DOI 10.1007/978-3-319-15904-1_2

KwaZulu-Natal students. However, the study only considered life satisfaction in general and not student satisfaction with campus residence life specifically.

The purpose of this paper is to add to the international and South African body of literature by investigating the correlates of student satisfaction with the quality of their campus residence life, drawing on a sample of students enrolled at small university in South Africa. Various possible predictors are examined under the following groups: (i) residence milieu and characteristics, (ii) direct and indirect discrimination, (iii) perceptions of drug and alcohol issues in residence, (iv) safety, and (v) individual student characteristics.

The remainder of this paper is structured as follows: section "The determinants of quality of life for university students: A literature review" contains a literature review of QoL determinants among university students in general and also provides an overview of university residence life within the South African context. Section "The Rhodes University context and residence system" discusses the university and residence context. Section "The data" presents the data, while section "Econometric methods" contains the methods employed. Section "Results" discusses the empirical results, and section "Conclusion" concludes.

The Determinants of Quality of Life for University Students: A Literature Review

While there is a fair amount of literature investigating the determinants of QoL among university and college students (Chow 2005; Sirgy et al. 2007; Zullig et al. 2009), it is mostly found in developed country contexts. In addition, while sometimes including campus-based residences, existing research seldom focuses specifically on *university* QoL, as opposed to QoL in general (Sirgy et al. 2007).[1] This is despite the fact that it has long been accepted that activities and conditions outside the classroom (what Kuh (1995) called "the other curriculum") can contribute to academic success, as well as the achievement of other important outcomes, such as "social competence, autonomy, self-awareness, and appreciation of human diversity" (Kuh 1995:124). In interviews with senior students from 12 US universities, it was found that increased humanitarianism (defined as concern for the welfare of others) was largely the result of interactions with peers and, to a lesser extent, leadership responsibilities, engaged in outside of the formal curriculum (Kuh 1995). University residential systems are thus ideal environments in which to foster such extracurricular outcomes.

This argument is supported by a review of 141 empirical studies on the determinants of life satisfaction for children and adolescents (Proctor et al. 2009). The

[1] In this paper, the terms "satisfaction", "well-being", and "quality of life" are used synonymously, though it is recognised that these terms can be used separately as well.

study showed that, in addition to the factors one might expect, such as personality, physical health and exercise, motivation, family relationships and so on, the physical environment, including environmental quality, living in a safe area and a having a well maintained home, had a significant positive association with well-being. Moreover, positive life satisfaction was associated with a better ability to deal with stress (Proctor et al. 2009).

Investigating the relationship between academic performance and QoL amongst students at a Midwestern university, Rode et al. (2005) used the "integrated life" model, which proposes that performance is a function of various life domain satisfaction levels, in this case, leisure, family, university and housing. "Housing satisfaction" had a positive, but not statistically significant impact on overall life satisfaction, but students with higher levels of life satisfaction generally did better academically. Rode et al. (2005:430) conclude that the implications of the integrated life model are that "the life-satisfied student is one who feels able to blend school and social life, as well as to maintain strong relationships with family and friends." Similar findings on the positive relationship between QoL and academic achievement were reported by Chow (2005) in a Canadian study and Rodgers and Summers (2008), who investigated why black students who went to predominantly white higher educational institutions in the United States did less well than their white counterparts, even when they had higher school-level grade point averages.

A study of Canadian students included housing conditions, divided into "living environment" (defined as the physical condition of the residence) and "living arrangements" (defined as the people being lived with) as determinants of the life satisfaction of university students (Chow 2005). Both factors were found to be positive and statistically significant determinants of QoL, but effects were much smaller than factors like self-esteem, relationship with "significant other," and socioeconomic status.

The only other study to focus specifically on student satisfaction with campus housing was done by Amole (2009) at a Nigerian university. However, the study is not directly comparable with this one because it focused almost exclusively on functional variables related to the physical structure of the residences. For example, it was found that students living in a residence with a kitchenette and shorter corridors were more satisfied than students residing in residences without these amenities.

In South Africa, access and success in higher education institutions can be an important and productive way of overcoming the racial discrimination of the past and the ongoing economic segregation of the present (CHE 2010). Diversity can also have important social and educational outcomes, such as "greater learning, increased interpersonal competencies, greater self-confidence among students, fewer irrational prejudices, greater gains in critical thinking, and greater involvement in civic and community service" (Worthington et al. 2008:8). Gottfredson et al. (2008) report that both diversity in the classroom and more informal "contact diversity" in other campus activities were positively related to such factors as cognitive openness, positive attitudes towards equal opportunities and academic outcomes.

Models of the determinants of student satisfaction can include a wide variety of factors related to (i) *student attributes*, such as race, sex, sexual orientation, age, socioeconomic status, self-esteem, drug and alcohol use, learning style, academic achievement; and (ii) *institution attributes*, for example living or housing conditions, on-campus social spaces and leisure activities, racial/ethnic diversity, dominant culture and so on (Chow 2005; Sirgy et al. 2007). An investigation of the well-being of students in university residences will tend to include items from both categories.

Student Diversity and QoL

An important component of student satisfaction with Higher Education Institutions is a sense of being part of the community or of "belonging" (Worthington et al. 2008; Nunez 2009). In addition to QoL studies, there has been an increasing use of "campus climate" surveys, particularly in identifying and understanding the experiences of students whose sexual orientation, race, or gender may have resulted in subtle forms of discrimination. The findings of both types of studies are reported here.

Miller and Sujitparapitaya (2010) compared campus climate surveys over time at a public university on the West Coast of the US to determine whether campus climate changed as the institution became more racially diverse. In 1994, the university had 40 % white students, which had fallen to 28 % by 2006. Among other questions, students were asked whether they had experienced or witnessed forms of insensitive behaviour (including incidents of "microaggression"). Contrary to expectations, they found that students answering "yes" to this question increased from 42 % in 1994, to 45 % in 1999 and 47 % in 2006. The results may be partly explained by the increase in "minority" students, who were more likely to have experienced such discriminatory behaviour, but the researchers also suggest that increasing diversity can make people feel defensive and threatened, and thus more likely to become segregated and aggressive. The challenge in such situations is to create an environment that fosters cooperation and not competition, which is likely to require purposeful intervention, rather than the assumption that integration will happen automatically.

Vaccaro (2010) conducted a qualitative analysis of written responses to open-ended questions in a campus climate survey conducted at a predominantly white university. Her findings showed that, while the results of campus climate surveys may appear to be mostly positive when based on closed-ended question responses, further analysis of written comments may reveal underlying prejudice and hostility. Despite official reports that described the climate as "positive" and "accepting" (Vaccaro 2010:205), the research showed alarming amounts of racism and sexism, particularly amongst male students. Women and black students, as well as staff, reported feeling excluded (by the presence of a "good old boy" network), devalued, and even unsafe.

Zullig et al. (2009) reported that students at a largely white university in the mid-west USA generally reported good or high QoL. They found that average reported QoL did not differ significantly between gender, race or "year in school", but that white students had a higher average than other groups. Similarly, a study of senior students from 17 research universities in the USA, with more than 14,000 responses, found that, overall, gender and race were not significant determinants of satisfaction. However, some differences across and between race groups were found: for example, Asian American women reported higher levels of satisfaction than did men from the same race group (Einarson and Matier 2005). Also, while the Miller and Sujitparapitaya (2010) study did find evidence of a "chillier" campus climate for some groups, they did not find evidence that lower perceptions of campus climate were statistically significantly related to student performance or persistence.

Health, Drug Use and Alcohol

In addition to student attributes, student behaviour has also been shown to have an impact on quality of life. Vaez and Laflamme (2003) investigated the relationship between the self-reported QoL and health (including lifestyle issues such as alcohol consumption, smoking and physical activity) amongst first year university students in Sweden. An interesting finding is that while male students rated their health lower on average than women, men still have a higher reported QoL mean score than women (Vaez and Laflamme 2003).

Despite the fact that many university students drink heavily, there have been few studies investigating the impact of alcohol use and student quality of life directly, and findings are often mixed (Murphy et al. 2005). For example, in a Canadian longitudinal study, greater alcohol use was associated with higher subjective well-being (Molnar et al. 2009). Murphy et al. (2005) found that men and white students reported drinking more heavily than women and students of other race groups, indicating gender and racial differences in consumption patterns. However, they also found that the relationship between life satisfaction and alcohol use (drinks per week) was quadratic, rather than linear, suggesting that moderate drinking improved life satisfaction, while complete abstinence and heavy drinking did not.

In terms of gender differences, heavy drinking episodes (up to 4 per week) increased the self-rated social quality of life satisfaction for men. For women, there was a negative relationship between drinking and general life satisfaction. Alcohol related problems reduced life satisfaction across all groups (Murphy et al. 2005). This accords with the findings of Vaez and Laflamme (2003), who found that male students were more likely to engage in frequent drinking (more than 2–4 times a week) and high consumption (7–9 glasses) than female students. While a relatively small percentage of the Swedish students in the sample smoked (24 %), smokers were much more likely to be men than women students.

Campus Climate and University Residence Life in South Africa

In 2010, the South African Council on Higher Education (CHE) published a report on “Access and throughput in South African higher education” with three universities chosen as case studies. Among the issues discussed relating to student persistence and success was university residence life: the residence culture and resultant degree of social integration of students being seen as important factors either promoting or hindering academic success (CHE 2010:108):

> Residences build unity, a commonness of purpose. First-year students look up to their seniors, and find the support and encouragement that accrue from loyalty to the residence. Rural students find residences a crucial bridge to the complexities and uncertainties of a large research university.

The first case study was the University of Pretoria (UP), which is a historically Afrikaans university with approximately 50,000 students. The CHE (2010:108) report found that the dominance of Afrikaans culture in UP residences could alienate black students, although significant improvements have been made since the banning of initiation ceremonies. The growing number of black leaders amongst residence students and staff has also helped to make the residences more culturally inclusive. In terms of achieving academic success, the residence experience was found to be an extremely important factor.

The University of the Witwatersrand (Wits) is a large and historically white, research university. Although not specifically related to residences, the study found that there was a group of students who were open to, and accepting of, the “rules, codes, norms and standards” of Wits social and institutional life and who feel they “belong” (CHE 2010:83). A second group were those who rejected these norms and traditions, emphasizing diversity and difference, while a third group felt displaced and alienated in the Wits environment. In addition, even for those students who feel they “belong”, there appeared to be ongoing issues of race, English-language ability, and xenophobia, although some spaces were seen as open and available to all (CHE 2010:86).

The final case study was the University of the Western Cape (UWC), a formerly black university. Here, residence culture appears to be much more accommodating of social diversity, but equally important in shaping social relationships, since students living on campus reported socialising mainly with other students living in residence (CHE 2010). Some residences also provided academic support in the form of mentoring programs and study groups. Problems experienced by students appeared to be largely related to communal living, such as loud music and other noise, lack of recreational and shopping facilities on campus and hygiene in residences. However, an important additional concern was around safety, both at drinking establishments on campus (“the Barn”), as well as off-campus (Cape Town and surrounds). Perceptions of the lack of safety were of particular concern to women as was the violence related to homophobia and xenophobia. In conclusion, UWC residences seem to offer a much more open and friendly environment than those of UP, and, despite continuing evidence of segregation in student clubs and societies, have had some success in cutting across race, gender and class boundaries (CHE 2010).

The University of Cape Town (UCT) campus climate survey (UCT 2007) focused on staff perceptions, rather than those of students. Nevertheless, similar patterns were found, with white men giving the highest percentage of positive responses to questions relating to campus climate, followed by white women, while African and foreign women had the highest percentages of negative responses. The most frequently cited problems with working at UCT were lack of racial diversity amongst the staff and racial discrimination (UCT 2007).

The Rhodes University Context and Residence System

Rhodes University is the smallest South African University by far, with approximately 7,400 students studying in 6 different Faculties. Approximately 25 % of the student body is international, and 25 % are postgraduate. Academic and support staff number 1,200. Founded in 1905, the University was formerly for whites only, a practice of racial segregation which was voluntary until 1959, when it was formally legislated. From the mid-70s black students were admitted in steadily increasing numbers, with a massive acceleration after 1994 and the end of apartheid. Today it is multicultural, multilingual and multi-ethnic in terms of student demographics, and faces the need for immense social transformation. Over 50 % of all students at Rhodes live in one of the university's 50 residences, including almost all of the first year students. Residences vary in size, with an average number of around 70 students per residence.

Students are housed on the basis of gender, and there are no co-ed residences. Each Residence has a live-in Warden, who (in additional to a full day job), is employed to ensure that both social and infrastructural needs are met, and that appropriate communal living standards and discipline prevail, in accordance with the University's protocols. Wardens are assisted by subwardens, appointed from amongst the senior students in the residence, and elected House Committees also play an active leadership role on a voluntary basis.

Led by a new Vice Chancellor since 2006, the University has set transformation at the top of the agenda, and the Dean of Students Office has energetically pursued strategies to raise awareness about diversity-related issues, to change mindsets and recognise and celebrate the diversity of its community by encouraging respect for human dignity, human rights, equality, non-sexism and non-racialism', in order to become a "home for all". This determination to encourage free speech, eschew violence, promote frank inquiry and tolerance and to reject discrimination of any kind is reiterated in the University's new Equity Policy and described in its Mission Statement: Rhodes University undertakes to develop shared values that embrace basic human and civil rights; to acknowledge and be sensitive to the problems created by the legacy of apartheid, to reject all forms of unfair discrimination and to ensure that appropriate corrective measures are employed to redress past imbalances.

The Data

The data originate from the 2011 Quality of Residence Life Survey conducted among students residing in campus residences at Rhodes University. Completed anonymously on paper by a representative sample of students from all 50 campus residences, this survey contains 50 questions on a 5-point Likert-type scale ranging from "strongly disagree" to "strongly agree" and is primarily aimed at ascertaining levels of general satisfaction with residence-life characteristics and identifying problem areas needing attention. For ease of interpretation in the regression analysis, the 5-point variables were re-coded to three categories each: "Strongly disagree" and "disagree" were collapsed as "disagree", "neutral" remained as a category on its own, and "agree" and "strongly agree" were collapsed into "agree". Such re-coding was also necessary since sample sizes in many categories of the 5-point variables were too small for reliable statistical inference. Apart from residential characteristics, the survey also records some demographic information regarding gender and race.

Although the survey has been conducted since 2007, the 2011 survey was the first to include a question on overall satisfaction with the quality of residence life, which asks students: "Using a scale of 1 to 10, where 1 is totally dissatisfied and 10 is totally satisfied, how satisfied are you with your quality of residence life?" For ease of interpretation in the descriptive analysis, a score of 1–3 was coded as "low", 4–7 as "medium", and 8–10 as "high". The choice as to which questions to include as measures of residential characteristics and campus life were guided in part by the literature and knowledge of the local university context. Table 2.1 presents the sample summary statistics. The average reported level of residence-life satisfaction is 7.21, suggesting that students are on average very satisfied with the quality of the residence life conditions.

Econometric Methods

This paper employs analysis of variance (ANOVA) as well as cross-tabulations between residence-life satisfaction and individual characteristics in the descriptive analysis. Student satisfaction with residence life is treated as ordinal and as such an ordered probit model is estimated to investigate the determinants of satisfaction with campus residence life. Student residence-life satisfaction for the ith student is assumed to be a function of residence and campus characteristics and individual student characteristics. Formally:

$$y_i = f(X_i, P_i) \quad (2.1)$$

where y_i is the 10-point variable capturing satisfaction with quality of residence life, X_i is a $(k \times 1)$ vector of residence and campus characteristics, and P_i denotes a

Table 2.1 Summary statistics

Variable	Mean	S.D.	Min	Max
Satisfaction with quality of residence life	7.21	1.64	1	10
Comfortable discussing personal issues with Warden	3.53	1.14	1	5
Residence is sufficiently quiet for study or sleep	3.56	1.10	1	5
Academic achievements are valued in residence	4.04	0.91	1	5
House Committee makes positive contribution to residence	3.93	0.89	1	5
Feel safe walking on campus at night	3.79	1.04	1	5
The disciplinary system is applied consistently and fairly	3.64	0.98	1	5
House Warden is able to assist in case of an academic problem	3.56	0.94	1	5
There is a drug problem in the residence	2.01	1.08	1	5
Experienced sexism	1.33	0.68	1	5
Experienced racism	1.50	0.88	1	5
Experienced a xenophobic incident	1.47	0.85	1	5
Clear and effective communication regarding events, safety and university news	3.80	0.84	1	5
There is an alcohol problem in the residence	2.47	1.18	1	5
Conflict in the residence is quickly and effectively resolved	3.64	0.91	1	5
Safety precautions in the residence are sufficient	3.85	0.83	1	5
Witnessed a violent incident in the residence	1.82	1.03	1	5
Satisfied with cleanliness of the residence	3.52	1.13	1	5
Always lock the room when not in it	3.78	1.21	1	5
Regularly have to queue in dining hall for longer than 10 min	2.50	1.21	1	5
Students respect individuality and each other's differences in the residence	3.92	0.84	1	5
The residence is well-maintained	3.73	0.99	1	5
Witnessed an unpleasant incident in residence involving sexism	1.47	0.78	1	5
Witnessed an unpleasant incident in residence involving racism	1.59	0.92	1	5
Witnessed an unpleasant incident in residence involving xenophobia	1.51	0.81	1	5
Years in residence	1.88	0.99	1	9
Male	0.39	0.49	0	1
Black	0.52	0.50	0	1
Coloured	0.04	0.19	0	1
Asian	0.04	0.19	0	1
White	0.34	0.47	0	1

$(k \times 1)$ vector of individual student characteristics. The ordered probit model is specified as:

$$y_i = \delta X_i + \gamma P_i + \varepsilon_i \tag{2.2}$$

where δ and γ are vectors of unknown parameters and ε_i is a randomly distributed error term. From the ordered probit results, this paper predicts marginal effects for a satisfaction score of eight or higher. These marginal effects indicate the average probability of reporting a satisfaction level of eight or higher.

Results

Figure 2.1 plots mean levels of satisfaction across racial groups, with white students reporting the highest score and black students the lowest.[2] However, according to ANOVA results, reported average satisfaction with residence life is not significantly different across racial groups ($F = 1.47, df = 3, 2{,}146, p = 0.2207$). Figure 2.2 indicates that, relative to female students, satisfaction is higher among male students, and this difference is statistically significant ($F = 8.89$, $df = 1$, 2,220, $p < 0.05$). Cross-tabulations between residence-life satisfaction and the individual traits of sex and race are presented in Table 2.2. Satisfaction across racial groups is relatively evenly spread across the various levels of satisfaction, and as noted, these differences are not statistically significant. Residence-life satisfaction is slightly higher among male students. For instance, about 52.5 % of male students reported a high level of satisfaction compared to 45.5 % of female students. This difference is statistically significant ($p < 0.01$).

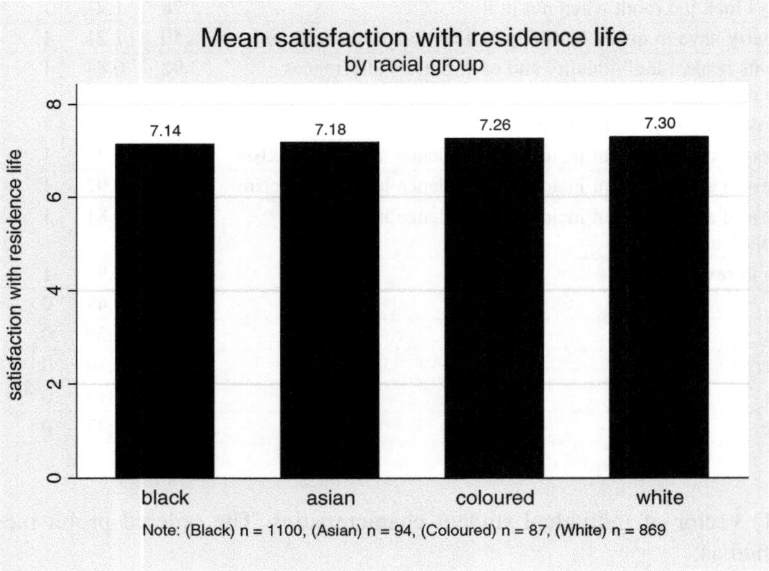

Fig. 2.1 Average residence-life satisfaction, by race

[2]Unless stated otherwise in section "Results", by "satisfaction" is meant "satisfaction with residence life".

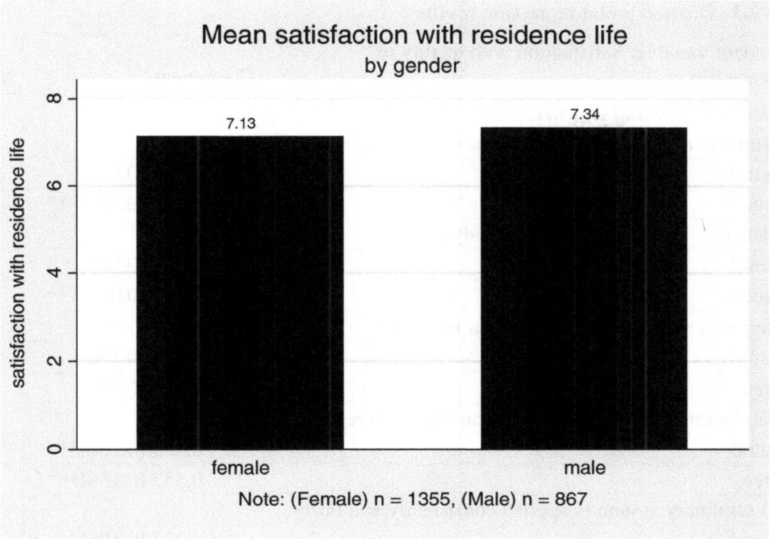

Fig. 2.2 Average residence-life satisfaction, by gender

Table 2.2 Satisfaction with residence life, by personal characteristics

	Satisfaction with quality of residence life			
Characteristics	Low	Medium	High	Total
Race				
Black	7.36 (n = 81)	46.55 (n = 512)	46.09 (n = 507)	100.0 (n = 1,100)
Asian	10.64 (n = 10)	40.43 (n = 38)	48.94 (n = 46)	100.0 (n = 94)
Coloured	3.45 (n = 3)	47.13 (n = 41)	49.43 (n = 43)	100.0 (n = 87)
White	5.98 (n = 52)	43.61 (n = 379)	50.40 (n = 438)	100.0 (n = 869)
Total	6.79 (n = 146)	45.12 (n = 970)	48.09 (n = 1,034)	100.0 (n = 2,150)
Pearson $\chi^2 = 8.24$ ($p = 0.221$)				
Gender				
Female	6.94 (n = 94)	47.53 (n = 644)	45.54 (n = 617)	100.0 (n = 1,355)
Male	6.34 (n = 55)	41.18 (n = 357)	52.48 (n = 455)	100.0 (n = 867)
Total	6.71 (n = 149)	45.05 (n = 1,001)	48.24 (n = 1,072)	100.0 (n = 2,222)
Pearson $\chi^2 = 10.30$ ($p < 0.01$)				

Note: "Low" denotes a satisfaction score of 1–4, "Medium" denotes a score of 5–7, and "High" denotes of score of 8–10

Table 2.3 contains the ordered probit regression results with the purpose of examining the predictors of student residence life satisfaction. The Wald χ^2 statistic ($p < 0.001$) indicates that the explanatory variables as a whole are statistically significant in explaining student residence-life satisfaction, with the Pseudo R^2 being roughly 13.3 %. Although this may seem low, such scores are common in cross-sectional studies. The remainder of this section discusses the regression findings by various sub-categories.

Table 2.3 Ordered probit regression results

Dependent variable: Satisfaction with quality of residence life	Coefficient	M.E.
Residence milieu and characteristics		
Comfortable discussing personal issues with Warden		
Neutral	0.034 [0.092]	0.011
Agree	0.388 [0.090]***	0.176
Residence is sufficiently quiet for study or sleep		
Neutral	0.116 [0.086]	0.087
Agree	0.412 [0.080]***	0.184
Academic achievements are valued in residence		
Neutral	−0.001 [0.146]	0.015
Agree	0.014 [0.139]	0.041
House Committee makes positive contribution to residence		
Neutral	0.405 [0.157]***	0.184
Agree	0.557 [0.156]***	0.216
The disciplinary system is applied consistently and fairly		
Neutral	0.223 [0.106]**	0.126
Agree	0.428 [0.104]***	0.212
House Warden is able to assist in case of an academic problem		
Neutral	0.210 [0.118]*	0.107
Agree	0.189 [0.121]	0.098
Clear and effective communication regarding events, safety and university news		
Neutral	0.046 [0.124]	0.083
Agree	0.078 [0.117]	0.089
Conflict in the residence is quickly and effectively resolved		
Neutral	0.019 [0.121]	0.026
Agree	0.274 [0.128]**	0.107
Witnessed a violent incident in the residence		
Neutral	−0.127 [0.087]	−0.012
Agree	−0.018 [0.110]	0.001
Satisfied with cleanliness of the residence		
Neutral	0.274 [0.082]***	0.120
Agree	0.338 [0.075]***	0.140
Regularly have to queue in dining hall for longer than 10 min		
Neutral	−0.146 [0.066]**	−0.034
Agree	−0.162 [0.072]**	−0.083
Students respect individuality and each other's differences in the residence		
Neutral	0.077 [0.148]	0.016
Agree	0.349 [0.144]**	0.121

(continued)

Table 2.3 (continued)

Dependent variable: Satisfaction with quality of residence life	Coefficient	M.E.
The residence is well-maintained		
Neutral	0.440 [0.104]***	0.174
Agree	0.792 [0.105]***	0.290
Discrimination		
Experienced: Sexism		
Neutral	0.061 [0.211]	0.028
Agree	0.400 [0.294]	0.178
Experienced: Racism		
Neutral	0.075 [0.133]	0.040
Agree	−0.024 [0.191]	−0.017
Experienced: Xenophobia		
Neutral	0.066 [0.166]	−0.022
Agree	0.070 [0.215]	0.003
Witnessed: Sexism		
Neutral	−0.226 [0.169]	−0.059
Agree	0.572 [0.197]***	0.267
Witnessed: Racism		
Neutral	−0.061 [0.141]	−0.020
Agree	−0.302 [0.153]**	−0.130
Witnessed: Xenophobia		
Neutral	−0.059 [0.157]	−0.067
Agree	0.052 [0.196]	0.002
Drugs and alcohol		
There is a drug problem in the residence		
Neutral	−0.186 [0.078]**	−0.062
Agree	−0.090 [0.124]	−0.011
There is an alcohol problem in the residence		
Neutral	−0.079 [0.066]	−0.006
Agree	−0.026 [0.088]	0.025
Campus and residence safety		
Feel safe walking on campus at night		
Neutral	−0.019 [0.098]	0.012
Agree	0.123 [0.092]	0.067
Safety precautions in the residence are sufficient		
Neutral	0.077 [0.138]	−0.029
Agree	0.142 [0.129]	0.007
Always lock the room when not in it		
Neutral	−0.074 [0.094]	−0.045
Agree	−0.140 [0.070]**	−0.062

(continued)

Table 2.3 (continued)

Dependent variable: Satisfaction with quality of residence life	Coefficient	M.E.
Individual characteristics		
Years in residence	−0.234 [0.104]**	−0.116
Years in residence squared	0.040 [0.021]*	0.021
Race		
Asian	0.073 [0.142]	−0.027
Coloured	0.010 [0.125]	0.046
White	0.005 [0.060]	0.027
Gender		
Male	0.025 [0.061]	−0.002
Pseudo R^2	0.1325	
Observations	1,566	
Wald χ^2	728.7***	
Log pseudolikelihood	−2510.7	

Note: $p < 0.001$***, $p < 0.05$**, $p < 0.10$*. Robust standard errors are reported in brackets. M.E. denotes the marginal effect that reflects the probability of reporting a satisfaction of eight or higher. For all answers ranging from "disagree" to "agree", omitted category is "disagree". For race, omitted group is "Black"; for gender, omitted group is "female"

Residence Milieu and Characteristics

In general, the characteristics of a particular residence, as well as the overall ambience of residence life, are important factors associated with campus residence-life satisfaction. Students who feel comfortable discussing personal problems with the residence Warden are more satisfied than those who do not ($p < 0.001$). The relationship is also quite strong: The former are 17.6 % more likely to report a satisfaction level of eight or higher. In contrast, there is not much evidence to suggest that student satisfaction is related to the House Warden's ability to assist with any particular academic issue. Although the perception of whether academic achievements are valued is not significantly related to residence-life satisfaction, a peaceful or quiet residence matters greatly for student well-being. Satisfaction levels are higher among those who feel that their residence is quiet enough for studying or sleeping relative to those that do not agree that this is the case ($p < 0.001$).

Having witnessed a violent incident in residence is not significantly associated with satisfaction with residence life; the same is true regarding the efficacy of communication regarding various news and events. A well-functioning House Committee as well as a fair disciplinary system are, however, very important for healthy student well-being. For instance, those who feel that the House Committee makes a positive contribution in the residence are more satisfied as opposed to those who perceive this not to be the case, and this association is quite strong ($p < 0.01$). Similarly, a perception that the disciplinary system is fair raises the likelihood of reporting a satisfaction level of eight or higher by about 21.2 % ($p < 0.001$). Both effective conflict resolution strategies within residence as well as mutual respect for students' individualism and differences are strongly associated with higher satisfaction with life in campus residence. For example, compared to students who do not feel that conflict resolution is adequate, those who reported satisfactory conflict resolution are 10.7 % more likely to possess a satisfaction level of eight or greater ($p < 0.05$). Likewise, students are significantly more satisfied if they believe that individuality and differences are respected ($p < 0.05$).

A clean and hygienic residence is positively associated with residence-life satisfaction, as students who feel that their residence is sufficiently clean, for instance, report significantly higher levels of satisfaction relative to students whose residences are not deemed acceptably clean ($p < 0.001$). Students do not like waiting for their food: Having to queue for longer than 10 min in the dining halls is negatively associated with student residence-life satisfaction ($p < 0.05$). Finally, the strongest relationship with residence satisfaction within the sub-category of residential characteristics is with maintenance. Students who feel that their residence is in good condition and well-maintained are 29.0 % more likely to report a satisfaction score of eight or greater than those that perceive that maintenance of their residence is poor ($p < 0.001$). This finding is supported by that of Chow (2005), who found a positive association between the physical condition of Canadian students' residences and student well-being.

Discrimination

Being a witness to discriminatory incidents is more strongly related to student satisfaction than actually directly experiencing a form of discrimination. Having witnessed incidents of sexism is positively associated with student well-being: Those having witnessed a sexist episode are 26.7 % more likely to report a satisfaction score of eight or higher when compared to those who have not witnessed such an incident ($p < 0.01$). While the latter finding may seem counterintuitive, it can be explained within the Rhodes University context of anti-sexism policies and awareness programmes. The University regularly has dedicated awareness campaigns focused on the elimination of sexism, with students also being encouraged to report sexist incidents. If students witness a sexist episode and subsequently report it, they may experience feelings of empowerment and gratification that serve to increase their perceived satisfaction with their residence life.

The opposite association is present if someone witnessed a racist incident. Students who have witnessed a racist episode are significantly less satisfied with their residence life as compared to students who have not witnessed such incidents ($p < 0.05$). This finding suggests that students are sensitive toward race-related incidents, which is reasonable given South Africa's long history of racial segregation and discrimination. Moreover, racial tensions have been shown to affect student QoL in the US (Miller and Sujitparapitaya 2010), for example, with race-related issues still being reported as problematic in South African universities (UCT 2007; CHE 2010) and this may also be the case in Rhodes University.

Drugs and Alcohol

Perceptions of an alcohol problem in residence seem to be negatively associated with student satisfaction, but only the coefficient of the neutral response is statistically significant. The practical significance of this finding is supported by Murphy et al. (2005) in that alcohol related problems are detrimental to student well-being. In the present case, the well-being of students who feel that alcohol abuse is an issue in their particular residence may be negatively affected through the actions of other students who drink frequently and heavily. There is no significant difference in satisfaction between students who agree and are neutral as to whether an alcohol problem exists ($p = 0.562$). Those that are neutral to the question about whether a drug problem exists in residence are less satisfied with their quality of residence life relative to students who disagree with the presence of drug issues ($p < 0.05$). Furthermore, there are no significant well-being differences among those who are neutral and who agree with the presence of a drug problem ($p = 0.457$).

Campus and Residence Safety

Perceptions of the degree of individual safety seem relatively important for student well-being. Those that feel safe on campus or perceive safety precautions in residence as adequate seem in general more satisfied with their residence life than students who do not feel safe or view the safety precautions as adequate. The coefficients measuring satisfaction differences with walking on campus are not statistically significant; the same is found for perceptions of safety precautions. However, post-estimation tests reveal that students who agree with feeling safe walking on campus are more satisfied than those who are neutral ($p < 0.05$). Also, those who lock their rooms when absent are significantly less satisfied compared to those that do not ($p < 0.10$), with the latter being about 6.2 % more likely to report a satisfaction score of eight or greater. Thus, feeling threatened by the possibility of theft or vandalism of personal possessions matters more for student satisfaction than feelings of general safety on campus and in residence. It should be noted, however, that the decision to lock their rooms may be linked to certain personality factors, which may also affect student satisfaction.

Individual Characteristics

The regression estimates indicate a significant non-linear relationship between the satisfaction with quality of residence life and the number of years living in residence. Student satisfaction with residence life does not differ significantly across either racial or sex groups. Further post-estimation equality of coefficient tests reveal no significant satisfaction differences between racial groups. The absence of such racial differences seem contrary to the environments at UP and UWC as noted earlier, where racial tensions often persist. These findings regarding sex and race in the present study are extremely encouraging, especially when viewed against the backdrop of the apartheid legacy and existing research.

Given the racial discrimination and historic marginalisation of women during the previous regime, we would expect to find substantial well-being differences between sex and racial groups. Furthermore, Ebrahim et al. (2013) find substantial discrepancies in subjective well-being across racial and gender groups in a study of the broader South Africa. It would thus seem that although we still observe well-being differences in the wider South African society between sex and race groups, such differences do not exist within the university environment under investigation (at least in terms of satisfaction with campus residence life). The findings from the present study regarding the absence of significant well-being differences between gender as well as racial groups are in accordance with research at US universities (Einarson and Matier 2005; Zullig et al. 2009).

Conclusion

The purpose of this study was to examine various correlates of student satisfaction with the quality of their campus residence life at South Africa's smallest university. Estimation of a basic ordered probit model reveals that student residence-life satisfaction is significantly associated with a range of direct and indirect factors, and as a whole emphasises the noted importance by previous research (Kuh 1995; Chow 2005) of campus residential factors in enhancing student well-being. A calm and serene residence environment is very important for high student satisfaction, in addition to well-maintained and clean residences. Important, especially within the context of South Africa's racially-divided past, is the absence of any substantial and statistically significant satisfaction differences between racial groups. Students value fairness in the application of disciplinary processes and the efficient resolution of conflict, as well as scope for individuality within residences as fostering greater residence-life satisfaction.

Indirect forms of discrimination are more important predictors of student well-being than are direct events of hate speech. For example, being a witness to a racist incident is detrimental to student satisfaction, while being the actual victim such an incident is not. The overall results with respect to hate speech or discrimination, whether experienced or witnessed, emphasise the continuing importance of efforts aimed at curbing such behaviour and in empowering students by urging them to report and speak out against all forms of discrimination or hate speech.

There is also some evidence to suggest that drug-related problems are detrimental to student well-being, and that perhaps some students are reluctant to divulge information in this regard. Residence-life satisfaction is lower among students who feel that they have to lock their dorm rooms when they are not present, implying that a perception of threat to personal property (by means of damage or theft, for example) is detrimental to student well-being. Perceptions of safety may also be linked to a student's personality, which itself could influence individual well-being. Improvements of security measures within campus residences, such as installing security cameras in residence hallways, are likely to benefit well-being by providing students with greater peace of mind.

Some limitations of this study should be noted. The cross-sectional nature of the data implies that only an analysis of associations can be performed and not causation. This also precludes any conclusions regarding the efficacy of certain university policies on student residence-life satisfaction. Moreover, the residence and campus characteristics analysed are based on each individual student's perception rather than actual characteristics: Students may perceive the same residence characteristic in different ways. Nevertheless, the findings from this paper have shown that residence factors and overall campus environment are important factors in enhancing student well-being. Careful planning and emphasis by universities on the internal and external situation of campus-based residences would be necessary in fostering healthy student well-being.

Acknowledgements We thank an anonymous referee for comments and suggestions. We also thank Alan Collins, Gavin Keeton, Geoff Antrobus, and participants at the 11th Conference of the International Society for Quality of Life Studies during 1–4 November 2012 in Venice, Italy, for helpful discussions and suggestions. The financial support of Economic Research Southern Africa (ERSA) is acknowledged.

References

Amole, D. (2009). Residential satisfaction in students' housing. *Journal of Environmental Psychology, 29*, 76–85.

CHE. (2010). *Access and throughput in South African Higher Education: Three case studies.* South African Council on Higher Education. www.che.ac.za/documents/d000206/. Accessed 21 Nov 2011.

Chow, H. (2005). Life satisfaction among university students in a Canadian prairie city: A multivariate analysis. *Social Indicators Research, 70*, 139–150.

Ebrahim, A., Botha, F., & Snowball, J. (2013). Determinants of life satisfaction among race groups in South Africa. *Development Southern Africa, 30*(2), 168–185.

Einarson, M. K., & Matier, M. W. (2005). Exploring race differences in correlates in seniors' satisfaction with undergraduate education. *Research in Higher Education, 46*(6), 641–676.

Gottfredson, N. C., Panter, A. T., Daye, C. E., Wightman, L. F., Allen, W. A., & Deo, M. E. (2008). Does diversity at undergraduate institutions influence student outcomes? *Journal of Diversity in Higher Education, 1*, 80–94.

Kuh, G. (1995). The other curriculum: Out-of-class experiences associated with student learning and personal development. *Journal of Higher Education, 66*(2), 121–155.
Miller, B., & Sujitparapitaya, S. (2010). Campus climate in the twenty-first century: Estimating perceptions of discrimination at a racially mixed institution, 1994–2006. *New Directions for Institutional Research, 145*, 29–52.
Møller, V. (1996). Life satisfaction and expectations for the future in a sample of university students: A research note. *South African Journal of Sociology, 27*(1), 16–26.
Molner, D., Busseri, M., Perrier, C., & Sadava, S. (2009). A longitudinal examination of alcohol use and subjective well-being in an undergraduate sample. *Journal of Studies on Alcohol and Drugs, 70*(5), 704–713.
Murphy, J. G., McDevitt-Murphy, M. E., & Barnett, N. P. (2005). Drink and be merry? Gender, life satisfaction and alcohol consumption among college students. *Psychology of Addictive Behaviors, 19*(2), 184–191.
Nunez, A. M. (2009). A critical paradox? Predictors of Latino students' sense of belonging in college. *Journal of Diversity in Higher Education, 2*(1), 46–61.
Prieto-Flores, M.-E., Fernandez-Majoralas, G., Forjaz, M. J., Rojo-Perez, F., & Martinez-Martin, P. (2011). Residential satisfaction, sense of belonging and loneliness among older adults living in the community and in care facilities. *Health and Place, 17*, 1183–1190.
Proctor, C., Linley, P., & Maltby, J. (2009). Youth life satisfaction: A review of the literature. *Journal of Happiness Studies, 10*, 583–630.
Rode, J., Arthuad-Day, M., Mooney, C., Near, J., Bladwin, T., Bommer, W., & Rubin, R. (2005). Life satisfaction and student performance. *Academy of Management Learning and Education, 4*(4), 421–433.
Rodgers, K. A., & Summers, J. J. (2008). African American students are predominantly white institutions: A motivational and self-systems approach to understanding retention. *Educational Psychology Review, 20*(2), 171–190.
Rojo-Perez, F., Fernandez-Majoralas, G., Rivera, F. E. P., & Rojo-Abuin, J. M. (2001). Age in place: Predictors of the residential satisfaction of elderly. *Social Indicators Research, 54*, 173–208.
Sirgy, M., Grzeskowiak, S., & Rahtz, D. (2007). Quality of college life of students: Developing and validating a measure of well-being. *Social Indicators Research, 80*, 343–360.
UCT. (2007). *University of Cape Town: Institutional Climate Survey Report 2007*. http://www.uct.ac.za/downloads/uct.ac.za/about/introducing/transformation/reports/institclimatesurvey07.pdf. Accessed 24 Nov 2011.
Vaccaro, A. (2010). What lies beneath seemingly positive campus climate results: Institutional sexism, racism, and male hostility towards equity initiatives and liberal bias. *Equity and Excellence in Education, 43*(2), 202–215.
Vaez, M., & Laflamme, L. (2003). Health behaviors, self-rated health, and quality of life: A study among first-year Swedish university students. *Journal of American College Health, 51*(4), 156–162.
Worthington, R. L., Navarro, R. L., Loewy, M., & Hart, J. (2008). Color-blind racial attitudes, social dominance orientation, racial-ethnic group membership and college students' perceptions of campus climate. *Journal of Diversity in Higher Education, 1*(1), 8–19.
Zullig, K. J., Huebner, E. S., & Pun, S. M. (2009). Demographic correlates of domain-based life satisfaction reports of college students. *Journal of Happiness Studies, 10*(2), 229–238.

Chapter 3
Life on Social Housing Estates: Studying Housing Quality with an Ethnographic Approach

Livia Bruscaglioni, Erika Cellini, and Barbara Saracino

The Dimensions of Housing Quality

Housing hardship does not stem solely from the quality and the suitability of the dwelling; it also derives from the system of relationships with the surrounding environment, the management of communal and relational spaces, and the perception of personal circumstances and space. The quality of housing is therefore a complex concept with diverse dimensions, each of which can be decomposed into various indicators. This article analyses the concept of housing quality in a specific context: that of social housing estates (henceforth SHEs).

In the research reported in this article, we considered six interconnected dimensions: the legal dimension; economic sustainability; the structural characteristics of the accommodation and the building; the quality of urban life in the neighbourhood; the quality of relations among inhabitants, local authorities and institutions; and the quality of relations among neighbours. The first four dimensions have been thoroughly analysed in the literature (see, for example, Tosi 1994; Ricci 1997; Olagnero 1998; EuroFound 2006; Poggio 2009), and they perfectly matched our research context. The final two dimensions emerged from our fieldwork.

One of the main dimensions identified in the literature is the quality of the so-called 'legal right to housing'. This dimension concerned our inquiry mainly in

---

Although this paper is the result of a joint effort, sections "The dimensions of housing quality" and "The context and the method of the study" were written by Erika Cellini, sections "Structures and people" and "Sense of community and conflicts" were written by Barbara Saracino, sections "Relations in spaces", "The symbolic elements of space" and "'Incivilities' as signals of the relationship with the institutions" were written by Livia Bruscaglioni; the conclusions were written by the authors together.

L. Bruscaglioni (✉) • E. Cellini • B. Saracino
Department of Political and Social Sciences, University of Florence,
via delle Pandette 21, 50127 Firenze, Italy
e-mail: bruscaglionil@gmail.com; erika.cellini@unifi.it; barbara.saracino@gmail.com

F. Maggino (ed.), *A New Research Agenda for Improvements in Quality of Life*,
Social Indicators Research Series 57, DOI 10.1007/978-3-319-15904-1_3

regard to non-property ownership: that is, the different rental situations of the tenants of social housing (rent bands, minimum social rent, arrears), as well as the unlawful occupation of dwellings, which differentiate among their experiences. In Italian SHEs, moreover, there are numerous owner-occupied flats: these are former publicly-owned dwellings mortgaged or purchased following sales campaigns by the municipalities. In some cases, the owners are the former tenants, who therefore do not differ socio-economically from current ones. In other cases, the owners have purchased their apartments from those who previously mortgaged them. As a consequence, SHEs comprise very different situations.

Among the economic aspects of housing quality, of central importance is the economic sustainability of expenditure on the home: that is, the proportion of income spent on the dwelling and its maintenance. In the literature, this problem is denoted with the term 'affordability', and it concerns the relationship between the household's economic resources and the various components of the dwelling's costs (Tosi 1994; Olagnero 1998). As Poggio (2009, 274) points out, housing costs may cause impoverishment because they reduce the resources available to satisfy other needs. This is problem frequently found among the residents of public housing projects, even though rent is calculated according to household income. The difficulties of finding and keeping jobs, or the frequent reliance on only a social pension, may make some residents unable to pay their utilities bills, or to refurbish their flats when they are in a poor state of repair. This increases housing hardship through the loss of services or the persistence of structural problems in the dwelling.

The dimensions that, according to Tosi (1994), define 'traditional' housing hardship are those that concern the structural characteristics of dwellings and buildings:

(a) adequacy of the dwelling with respect to the presence or absence of essential services (a telephone line, sanitary installations, hot running water, central heating). Essential services are usually guaranteed in public residential housing; they are therefore valid indicators of housing quality, and the absence of only one of them indicates a decidedly deprived state of housing;
(b) adequacy of the dwelling with respect to the occupiers' needs in terms of personal space and cohabitation (number of rooms per occupant, square metres per occupant);
(c) the dwelling's suitability in terms of the age of the building and its state of repair. For SHEs, it is important to evaluate characteristics relative to ordinary and extraordinary renovation, because its presence or absence may significantly change housing quality for residents.

Also the quality of urban life in the neighbourhood is considered an important dimension of housing quality (EuroFound 2006, 59). The main indicators of this dimension relate to four sub-dimensions: ecological aspects concerning the presence or the quality of green areas and pollution levels; the quality of public spaces; the presence of services and shops, transport and infrastructure; the district's links with the other parts of the city; personal safety with respect to petty crime or the perception of it.

A fifth dimension relates to relations between residents and the institutions mainly concerned with SHEs: the public agencies that allocate dwellings and manage the public housing stock. Those who wish to live in a social housing project, or already do so, must necessarily deal with these agencies. The type and quality of relations with depend on several factors with differing levels of complexity: housing policies, the economic resources made available, the procedures adopted and their level of bureaucratization, the attitudes of the public agencies towards citizens, the behaviour of individual staff and users, and the presence of forms of self-management by tenants that can facilitate relations with the public housing authority.

The last, but not least important, dimension relates to the quality of the social relations among neighbours: that is, localized social relations which include the neighbourhood but are not confined to it: what Bagnasco (1999) terms 'proximity-based relations'. By now consolidated in the debate on social exclusion is a conception of deprivation as not only socio-economic but also, if not especially, relational (Sen 1985). Analysing individual isolation or the quantity of a person's social relations therefore makes it possible to determine the degree of participation in the various levels of society (Negri and Saraceno 2000). Relations among neighbours have altered as a consequence of changes in the structure of the family and levels of population mobility. The neighbourhood as "instance sociétale de proximité" (Genestier 1999) may have lost centrality in the lives of the inhabitants of contemporary cities. In social housing projects, the neighbourhood as a relational space is still important: SHEs are largely inhabited by people with reduced mobility – children, the elderly, disabled persons, and members of marginalized groups – who pursue many spheres of their lives in those settings (Authier et al. 2007) and whose social networks are restricted to them (Fischer 1982).

The semantic sphere of housing quality includes many other aspects, which overlap with the more general idea of the quality of life related to economic resources, employment levels, socio-cultural and health conditions, and psycho-physical well-being. All these dimensions can also be considered simultaneously as factors that produce housing hardship. "The life-quality of a resident of a decayed neighbourhood is the result of numerous interconnected dimensions not reducible merely to refurbishing his or her home" (Sclavi et al. 2002, 115). The literature states that "the quality of housing, the type of building, and the place where one lives reflect the structure of inequalities in society" (Poggio 2009, 275), and that housing hardship can itself be an indicator of other types of "social hardship, in particular the lack of economic and citizenship resources that is created in the economic system and which is manifest – although not exclusively – in housing privation" (Olagnero 1998, 48). The housing quality level therefore reflects the quality of life in general: housing hardship is indicative of the existence of a social risk "that individuals and family groups run not only as *occupiers* of accommodation or as residents of an area, but also as individuals already *socially excluded* (by exit or non-entry) from the social groups that govern the process of entering and remaining within the system" (Olagnero 1998, 51). These are individuals who already belong to vulnerable social groups (Zajczyk et al. 2005; Atkinson et al. 2002).

The Context and the Method of the Study

The concept of housing quality, and its various aspects, was studied by the research group on public housing estates in Livorno, a city of central Italy and the most important port in the region of Tuscany.

The history of public residential housing in Livorno is closely associated not only with issues that relate to the urban development of the city throughout the twentieth century, but also with its social and cultural identity and socio-economic profile. The residential public housing neighbourhoods built since the beginning of the nineteenth century have accompanied the development and social history of the city and the transformations in its productive and economic fabric (Bortolotti 1967; Pierini 2001). Notwithstanding the fact that the size of the property portfolio has been reduced through sales, the city's residential public housing areas are still the foundation of its structure, and they make it the most 'public' city in Tuscany, with social housing representing nearly 8 % of the total number of dwellings (compared with approximately 3 % in Tuscany and Italy overall).[1] This is a percentage that approaches European levels, with regard to which Italy as a whole occupies one of the bottom places (Eurostat 2010).

In the first phase of the research, the concept of housing quality was studied using various investigative strategies and tools: the historical reconstruction of areas of residential public housing and the laws applying to it; analysis of statistical data produced by official sources (especially Casalp – the agency that manages public housing in Livorno – the municipality, and the regional administration); and interviews conducted with a number of key informants. Based on these studies, we chose two areas with a large amount of residential public housing – Barriera Garibaldi and La Leccia – where we could investigate our research topic in more detail using an ethnographic approach.

We used the immersion method. This a technique characteristic of ethnographic research whereby the researcher joins a community and observes it 'from within', taking part in its life and applying the principle of non-separateness between those who study and those who are studied.

We lived in Livorno from September 2011 to August 2012, after a brief search for a flat that would enable the members of our group to avoid having to commute from Florence, but rather to experience life in the area and the daily lives of its inhabitants at all times of the day, to interact with them, to establish relationships, and to become a recognizable presence. At Barriera Garibaldi the search for a flat was the initial phase of access to the field assisted in particular by the barman at

[1] The data refer to 2010, and are our own calculations tables provided by the *Agenzia del Territorio* (2011), the Regione Toscana (2012, 95) and Casalp – Casa Livorno e Provincia S.p.A. – which has managed the public residential housing portfolio of the Province of Livorno since 2004.

the *Circolo ARCI*[2] located in the heart of the neighbourhood. Our relationship with the barman – who assumed the classic role of a 'guarantor' (Gobo 2001, 93–94) – enabled us to meet most of the habitués of the Circolo, to interview many of them informally and some of them formally, and to have the Circolo become a privileged observation point for the research group, at least initially. At La Leccia the president of the local social centre (a centre where the Municipality organises activities for older inhabitants of the area) assumed the role of 'garantor' and let us to contact and interview many residents.

Immersion involves the use of diverse research tools. In our case, during the year spent in the field, we decided:

- to collect already-existing documentary material on Livorno's neighbourhoods: to consult documents and books on the local context and city planning reports, among them urban renewal plans; to collect newspaper articles on life in the two neighbourhoods.
- to collect audio and video materials both a simple method to record information and a way to report the research results.
- to conduct observation – the method whereby the researcher observes and records ongoing events and behaviours without deliberately eliciting them with verbal or behavioural prompts (Cellini 2008, 16–17), and the settings in which they occur. In particular, we chose to use overt observation. We therefore declared our identities and the aims of our research to all the residents with whom we came into contact. Overt observation enabled us constantly to share the assumptions and conduct of the research; to be present in different social situations; to flank observation with other information-gathering techniques; and to alternate the fieldwork with brief periods of deskwork.
- to carry out semi-structured interviews with key informants, and in-depth interviews eliciting the life histories of the residents of the neighbourhoods selected for analysis (Atkinson 1998; Bichi 2007).[3] We decided to use life histories rather than interviews focused on housing quality because of the semantic nature of the concept. As said, the quality of housing is not solely associated with the quality of the accommodation in the strict sense. Moreover, life histories allow the

[2] The ARCI is the Italian Recreation and Cultural Association, and is one of the most important in the country. It was created in the 1950s with the aim of uniting the clubs, social centres ("*case del Popolo*"), and mutual assistance societies ("*società di mutuo soccorso*") expressing democratic and anti-fascist ideals. ARCI clubs are still today places where people gather, above all in the regions of central Italy that typified the so-called 'Red' sub-culture (Trigilia 1983), for political as well as recreational and cultural social activities. Many of them housed local branches of the Italian Communist Party, and these days they host the local offices of the left or centre-left parties.

[3] The sample for life histories was constructed based on the criteria of social representativeness, taking emerging theory, previous knowledge and the specificity of the field into account. The main strategy was the maximization of diversity. The operating principle was that of constructing subsets: the research group divided the populations of the two districts into subgroups based on both individual and context dimensions: age and sex of the individual, the year of settlement in the area, and the building of residence.

interviewees' dimensions of meaning to emerge without the application of conceptual categories preconstituted by the researcher, in accordance with the principles of grounded approach (Glaser and Strauss 1967).

By living in the neighbourhood with the residents, we were able to obtain narratives on the various dimensions of housing quality and the related concepts as they were perceived, recounted, and experienced by the social actors themselves, and to understand the significance of their homes for the respondents – actions and interactions, concrete facts, and daily complexities: all the elements that make up the way of life of actors (individuals, families, and small groups) in working-class areas. Citing La Cecla (2005, 3), we might say that there is a specific cultural modality of habitation that consists of the "perception, definition, and use of a space that only those who belong to it as residents can truly possess".

The positive aspects of a residence depend not only on its characteristics but also on its effect on people's lives. The quality of housing cannot be captured by statistical data alone. In order to be fully understood, information on the structural quality of accommodation and buildings and the sociographic characteristics of the tenants must be supplemented with the meanings given to them by the latter. Figures on the state of disrepair of dwellings do not recount the frustration of the people who live in them. Stating the small size of a flat in terms of square metres does not convey the difficulty of living in cramped conditions. The number of elderly people living alone does not tell the story of their loneliness.

To be noted is that there were frequently in group in the field.[4] Our experience was therefore distinct from that of classic studies in which the ethnographer alone immerses him/herself in the field,[5] particularly in activities relative to access to the field, immersion in it, note-taking, and interpreting the information gathered.

As members of a group, we were able to handle our solitude, not to feel out of place, and not to suffer significant exclusion from the context. Each member of the group, with his or her own characteristics, got to know different people and gained their trust; but as in a game of mirrors, they also reflected this trust on to the others. It could be said that, in practice, it was as though each of us acted as the 'guarantor' for the others.

Carrying out our research in a team reduced the problem of tiredness, and helped us overcome emotional problems, offering psychological support above all at times when there was an accumulation of stories of life problems, or when minor accidents occurred. The fact that there were in group in the field fostered polysemy in our interpretation of the information gathered (Colombo and Navarini 1999). Even when we had been simultaneously present in the same situation, our initial

---

[4] During the research time the following people have been members of the research group: Serena Borgi, Fabrizio Bruno, Livia Bruscaglioni, Erika Cellini, Rosa Di Gioia, Gianluca La Bruna, Valentina Pappalardo, Elisa Proietti, Dario Raspanti, Barbara Saracino, and Barbara Vidili.

[5] Although ethnography is conceived in the collective imagination as a solitary activity, a good deal of sociological and anthropological research is often the result of teamwork (Douglas 1976; Salzman 1989).

interpretations were not always the same. Observation is influenced by the researcher's conceptual categories, life experiences, and theoretical knowledge. Through our 'ethnographic performance' (Sacchetti 2012), we were almost always able to arrive at shared, inter-subjective interpretations.

Barriera Garibaldi and La Leccia – the two areas that we investigated using the ethnographic approach – are very different from each other according to a number of criteria related to the dimensions of housing quality considered. Section "Structures and people" compares the two districts on the basis of certain structural characteristics of the housing and the buildings, the legal dimension, economic sustainability, and the quality of urban life in the neighbourhood. Section "Relations in spaces" applies an interpretative frame based on the ties between persons and spaces to compare other aspects of the quality of urban life in the neighbourhood, the quality of relations among residents, local authorities and institutions, and the quality of relations among neighbours.

Structures and People

The construction of Barriera Garibaldi began in the 1930s during the Fascist era, and it was completed in the years following the Second World War. The area is located in the north-east of Livorno, between the port and the railway station, in a working-class area of the city, close to other public housing areas with evocative names such as Shangay and Corea. It was once outside the city centre, but today it is part of the main axes of the city.

The Leccia public housing project, built in the early 1980s, is situated in the south-eastern zone of Livorno, distant from the city centre. The neighbourhood lies outside the city's main transit routes and is consequently seldom traversed by non-residents.

Barriera Garibaldi currently consists of 44 residential public housing buildings arranged around six courtyards, which face on to the main square and two main streets. 722 residences are managed by Casalp (representing 12 % of the public housing stock in Livorno) for a total of 1,561 inhabitants (11 % of the total of SHE residents).

The La Leccia social housing project consists of three blocks: the so-called '*palazzi grigi*' (built with prefabricated materials in response to a housing emergency with a view to their future demolition), the so-called '*palazzi rossi*', and the buildings in Via Guadalajara. There are 455 flats in these buildings (7.5 % of the total housing stock managed by Casalp) and 1,057 people live in them (8 % of the total SHE residents in Livorno).[6]

In the case of Barriera Garibaldi, the Fascist regime decided that the working class must be moved out of the city centre, and that the buildings should take the

[6] The data cited in this section are own calculations on matrices supplied by Casalp.

form of large tenements with internal courtyards, so that hostility against the regime could be controlled. On walking through the area, one sees Foucault's (2001) reflections in concrete form: space is fundamental for every exercise of power, and architecture is a technical manifestation of power. When the regime constructed the buildings, it paid more attention to their external monumental aspect (the four original blocks spell out the word 'DUCE') than it did to the interior. Just like dwellings at the beginning of the industrial revolution, many of the flats do not have two outlooks, and they are small and of poor quality.

The situation in Barriera Garibaldi is today the most problematic of the various public housing areas in Livorno: the state of repair of many buildings is poor (according to Casalp's classification, only 31 % of the houses are 'normal'), 40 % of the flats have less than 45 m^2 of floor space.

Over the years, there have been few interventions in Barriera Garibaldi, owing to political decisions, reductions in funding, and managerial incompetence. In recent years, the economic resources available have been focused on the recovery plan for the other northern areas of the city. While we were in the field, a recovery plan was also approved for Barriera Garibaldi, but it has begun slowly, and will take many years to carry out. Some of the buildings and residences are today in very poor condition: structural problems such as the lack of lifts, subsiding floors, water leaks, widespread damp, and sub-standard bathrooms make daily life unsustainable.

At La Leccia, even though according to the Casalp classification there are no sub-standard dwellings, and the flats are larger than those of Barriera Garibaldi, the poor quality of the buildings (constructed with the massive use of prefabricated materials) is such to cause major problems – as also evidenced by the interviews with the residents.[7]

La Leccia has a number of features that distinguish if from the other SHEs in Livorno: for instance, its mixed public/private character. To understand these features, it should be borne in mind that La Leccia was originally designed in response to a housing emergency in the city, but it was also intended to be an experiment. The last large-scale public housing project before La Leccia, in fact, had been in the adjacent district of Salviano, where the strong concentration of people at risk of social marginality due to the housing emergency had created conflicts with the existing social fabric. To obviate the problems at Salviano, La Leccia was conceived as a combination of publicly- and privately-owned dwellings. Today La Leccia takes the form of a 'mixed' neighbourhood in which social housing is embedded within a larger context of private properties.

While the early recipients of public housing were working class, successive housing laws have introduced gradual changes into the social conditions of the

[7] I did the work, and the rain kept coming into the flat [. . .] Everything was damp, because the window frames weren't fitted properly [. . .] so we turned the windows round. For instance, the windows in the living room and the kitchen both opened towards the door. . . so the work had been shoddy, I don't know who could have made them. Also the builder, the surveyor, the engineer who designed these houses, I mean, they can't have studied very much (woman, 36–50 years old, resident for ten years).

residents. Tuscany Regional Law no. 96 of 1996 now uses assignment criteria to determine the applicants eligible for social housing. Among the requirements that make up the overall score for an applicant household are not only low income but also other socially relevant characteristics, such as the presence of a disabled or invalid person in the household, large numbers of children or a single parent, the unhealthy state of the current home, or being subject to eviction proceedings.

According to data from the City of Livorno Housing Department, very few flats become available in the city each year – around 30 – compared with the demand, which is over one thousand per every call for applications (the general preference list is valid for 2 years). For this reason, the applicants who obtain public housing are only those at the top of the waiting list, where the score awarded them is the sum of a number of problem issues. In 2012, the average rent – an indicator of the economic circumstances of a family because it is calculated on the basis of the household income – is 72 euros at Barriera Garibaldi and 122 euros at La Leccia; the percentage of single-parent families 15 % at Barriera Garibaldi and 8 % at La Leccia; the percentage of households with a disabled person is around 20 % in both districts.

Since the 1990s, the Tuscany regional administration also required that any flat of fewer than 35 m^2 that becomes available should no longer be assignable by drawing on the general waiting list. The Livorno city council has decided that this type of accommodation should be given to 'housing emergency' cases: that is, to persons not on the waiting list but who find themselves homeless due to eviction, return from rehabilitation communities, or release from psychiatric care.

Barriera Garibaldi is the neighbourhood with the highest percentage of flats allocated for emergency housing. At La Leccia, instead, the proportion is insignificant.[8] At Barriera Garibaldi this policy decision therefore brings into the neighbourhood many people whose past includes outright exclusion from housing and whose present includes unemployment or social and health problems sometimes taking the form of substance dependence. The low quality of housing in this neighbourhood from a structural viewpoint co-exists with, and is therefore additional to, other forms of deprivation (social, health, or employment), more than one of which frequently affects the same individual.

Barriera Garibaldi is a 'dense' area because of the high number of residences and residents, but also because of the large number of commercial businesses and services locally available to the residents. The neighbourhood is also well served by public transport, with links to the various key points in the city, for instance the administrative centre, the hospital, or the railway station. The residents can reach all of these places with a short walk or bus journey.

At La Leccia, there are few businesses in the neighbourhood, services are scant, and connections with the rest of the city are poorly developed. Public transport does not cover all routes to the other districts of the city, like those, for instance, close to the sea.

[8] According to data issued by the City of Livorno Housing Department relative to the allocation of emergency accommodation between 2006 and 2010, out of a total of 99 dwellings, 43 were assigned to Barriera Garibaldi and only one to La Leccia.

The neighbourhood was built on an agricultural land in a very short period of time. Its planned layout is the so-called 'dormitory' area with prefabricated houses. Its characteristics reflects the historic image of the Italian urban hinterland: lack of public (and private) services, socio-economic vulnerability of its inhabitants, inappropriate construction typologies, geographical distance from the urban centre, and poor integration with the city.

Relations in Spaces

Simmel (1908) defines space as the possibility of being-together, in that reciprocal action turns empty space into something solid for those who experience it: hence, action fills space insofar as space makes it possible. The connection between persons and spaces can be considered bilateral and two-directional: human actions and relations jointly create and transform spaces while they are in turn simultaneously created and transformed by them (D'Aloisio 2011, 173–174).

The sense of space is the result of particular social relations. The inhabitants of a place appropriate the space available to them and transform it into a set of collectively recognized places which are subject to shared social practices – that is, practices endowed with a collective sense and produced by a "localized culture" (Augé 1992, 48).

A space can have functions, uses, and practices. A space's functions – usually imagined by planners – concern the roles that it must perform in the general organization of the neighbourhood and the city. The uses made of a space by the inhabitants relate to the physical and material aspects of residence and the connected activities. Practices relate the physical and material dimensions to the cultural and symbolic ones inhering in the ways in which spaces are concretely inhabited and experienced (Cellamare 2011). The idea that a space conceived and designed in a particular way must perform functions useful for those who use it sometimes becomes of secondary importance if the meaning that people attach to it suggests alternative uses or non-uses.

In SHEs, spaces derive from the interaction between the material forces that produce them and the individuals who live in them, give them meaning, and transform them. More than others, the residents of SHEs live in a particular frame (Goffman 1974) and with an urban 'strategy' imposed by specific modes of codification and use. The functions are defined by the institutions, and the spaces are assigned to the inhabitants. In these contexts, the residents can adopt 'tactics': they can make the spaces their own, modifying them with use and individual and collective practices (De Certeau 1990). But they can only do so within certain limits: renovations, for instance, are decided by the institutions, often without involving the inhabitants.

According to Gasparini (2000, 209–210), the symbolic value of places is of composite nature: it can be related not only to the experience of social and interpersonal relations, but also to the history of the group and the individual, to the accumulation of facts that are culturally interpreted, emotionally experienced, invariable (habit) or traumatic and unique. On studying the processes of space appropriation, it is possible to reconstruct the memory and the collective history of places and the groups that live in them (Halbwacks 1968). Urban symbolism contributes to structuring the processes which determine the identity of the inhabitants (Mela 1999, 148) and their sense of local belonging. People live and act in spaces; they orient themselves according to spaces; they construct and redefine identity within and through spaces. But they also modify spaces by adapting them to their needs and identities.

The Symbolic Elements of Space

If one considers the spatial organization of a city and its districts as connoted by strong symbolic values tied to aesthetic and cultural meanings and their social function of constructing a sense of belonging (Gasparini 2000), the presence or absence of a 'centre' – a square as the symbolic place *par excellence* – is an important factor in understanding the quality of life in a neighbourhood.

La Leccia was the first example of a peripheral neighbourhood in Livorno with no meeting places like squares and pedestrian areas and few neighbourhood shops: there is only one shopping centre.

La Leccia is characterized by the lack of a 'centre' and a 'square', and by the presence of empty spaces with no function foreseen for them at the planning stage; spaces which do not encourage uses and practices by the local residents and therefore the accumulation of social routines, or of the emotionally important events that imbue places with symbolic value (Gasparini 2000). These are areas to which the planners originally assigned no function, and which over time have not seen practices of spontaneous meaning attribution by the inhabitants.

Two a-functional areas in particular strike one's attention in the neighbourhood's geography. The first is a public space in front of the shopping centre. Despite various proposals for its re-modelling over the years, still today this broad area is devoid of a function. The second example is a private space situated to the interior of one of the housing blocks.

> It's a sort of large courtyard with an artificial hillock in the middle made when they constructed the buildings. According to one of the residents, it should be levelled, they should put benches there. Instead, it has not function apart from dog-walking. The internal space is considered 'private', so that maintenance of the lighting is at the expense of the residents. If a lamp-post (I saw one lying on the ground) breaks, it's not fixed by the residents because they don't want to spend the money. The inner space of the buildings is thus neglected. In effect, the impression is one of a neglected and 'functionless' space (ethnographic note 02.20.2012).

The two above-mentioned areas exemplify cases in which the residents, faced with spaces whose function was not made explicit at the design stage, have not set about converting them into collectively recognized places – that is locus of shared social practices. In the case of the public space in front of the shopping centre, it was only used by the residents to walk from one place (the shopping centre) to another (the bus stop); a use perceived by some elderly residents as dangerous given the place's state of neglect.

To use Lynch's terms (1960), in la Leccia, we find neither the 'nodes' nor the 'landmarks' that are clearly visible in Barriera Garibaldi.

Barriera Garibaldi is the official name of the neighbourhood and its main square, but the residents prefer to use the term 'La Guglia' to indicate where they live. La Guglia is the name of the obelisk in the square, but it is used to refer to the entire district because of the symbolic importance given by the residents to the monument

Barriera Garibaldi Square may be considered a *node* because it is a convergence point, a strategic location for individuals' spatial behaviour; it is the place where relationships assume a verbal and physical representation. Their landmarks, the reference points represented by easily-identifiable physical elements, are the obelisk and the so-called 'tree of the dead birds'[9] for the 'established', the palm trees and the corner in front of the bar for the 'outsiders'.

In regard to the 'La Guglia' neighbourhood, it is productive to use Elias's conceptual dichotomy between the *established* and *outsiders* (Elias and Scotson 1994). In the course of our ethnographic research in Barriera Garibaldi, we identified the 'established' as the oldest residents, those who had always lived in the neighbourhood, in homes assigned to their families before the war or immediately afterwards. And we identified three types of *outsiders* with respect to the established residents: foreigners, 'multi-problem' families (as we term them), and drug addicts (Cellini and Saracino 2013).[10]

Despite the conflict between these groups (see the following sections), for all of them La Guglia is a place where intense relationships are formed, where there is solidarity and 'resistance' to life's difficulties and the forces of mass society that lead to breakdown and alienation, a place where they can find emotional and instrumental support, a place that gives them an identity, roots, and attachment, a place of memory and where shared social rules are created.

In particular, the elderly established men have very intense everyday relations in two places in Barriera Garibaldi Square, which have acquired meaning in the course of time. The function given by the designers to the 'tree of the dead birds' is to make the square more attractive, and the obelisk serves as a traffic divider and as a

---

[9] I don't know why, but they tell us that tree over there is called the tree of the dead birds and laugh. I ask them to tell me why, and they laugh and talk about their age and how they are close to death. In fact, they were referring to their genitalia, which no longer function. But I hadn't understood this properly... (ethnographic note, 09.22.2011).

[10] The use of Elias's categories and the description of outsiders as opposed to established people are based on the roles we took on the field. The way the research is conducted and the roles taken on by the researchers or assigned to them by social actors may lead to the construction of knowledge which is based on the perceptions and viewpoints of a specific group of social actors, or on what the researcher has experienced most intensely on the field. Due to roles we assumed on the field, and to the centrality of the established people in the life of the area, the perspective of the latter was predominant, but not exclusive, in our interpretive process.

monument. Both are used by the inhabitants as benches. Over time, both places (one in the morning before lunch, and the other in the evening before dinner) have become spaces for old friends, where they talk, complain, make fun of each other, argue, and check on the neighbourhood and the people that frequent it. The way in which they use these spaces is made possible by the social and cultural constructs implicit in the division of gender roles. The women look after the home and prepare lunch or dinner, so that the men can linger in the square until their meals are ready. The wives know where to find their husbands: they go to the window, they see them, and they call them home (Cellini and Saracino 2013).

The older women mix to a lesser extent: they stay at home or do the shopping in the many shops in the neighbourhood or close to it. Originally, they used to get together on chairs in the courtyard, and the courtyard was a gathering-place where they could share their problems. Today, the courtyards no longer have this role, at least not as much as they did before.

> There where my mum is, they've known each other for fifty years! Everyone knows everything about everyone there ... there aren't many recent arrivals [...] they are all the original residents, yeah, they're the original families [...] my mum was born there! My granny lived there. She was a widow ... then she met my granddad .... they had my mum late, granny was 47 and granddad was 57 [...] so she's practically lived there for ever, she never... and then there wouldn't even be a way to move out [...] absolutely not! [...] she's really attached to the place [...] in the summer, they go, they all take their folding chairs, and go down [...] they play cards [laughs], it's great to see them, there's really an.. an interaction among them that's just like a family! [...] they chat, they bicker [...] if one of them has a problem, she goes to see someone, who goes to see someone else[...] but if you take this building for example, these things don't exist (woman, aged 51–66, born in the neighbourhood).

'Incivilities' as Signals of the Relationship with the Institutions

The presence of incivility – defined as a lack of standard of care and maintenance of the territory (environmental incivility) or a violation of standards in the sharing of public spaces (social incivility) – is a further element that should be taken into account when seeking to understand the quality of urban life in a neighbourhood, as well as the relations among the residents, and those between the residents and the institutions.

The so-called "incivility hypothesis" (Chiesi 2004, 133) links the perception of elements of incivility by residents to the creation of a sense of unease and to an increase in demands for security. According to this model, a persistent perception of signs of incivility may give rise to a sense of unease, to a retreat from public spaces, to a sense of having been abandoned by the institutions which protect the territory, and finally to a weakening of social ties and sense of community. The perception of incivilities may modify the meanings of places, the opportunities that they can offer, and the sense of belonging.

In the context of La Leccia, the perception of incivilities and of solitude and isolation were recurrent topics in the interviews. The perception of isolation and distance mainly concerned the relationship with the local institutions: the municipality and Casalp. Incivilities were seen not so much as signs of deviant behaviour as evidence of a distance from the institutions.

This sense of malaise was due to the perception of signs of incivility in public spaces, and to the feeling of living in a neighbourhood abandoned by the institutions, which did little work on buildings intended to be provisional. The signs of incivility became themselves signs of distress. As key informants we collected interviews with local administrators, like the president of the *Consiglio di Zona* (District Council). This was the local branch of the municipal administration, and it should have been the body closest to the community. The District Council has among its objectives to collect opinions on life in the district from residents.

> This neighbourhood here is a bit abandoned . . . it's a place where, let's say . . . these should have been temporary houses, then they should have been abolished, torn down, but instead they're still normal. What do the people here ask for? That the institutions should be present. If in this field where people take their dogs and where people are happy to come, the grass is fifty centimetres high, how do we see it? We feel uneasy! But this perception starts when the neighbourhood is all dark, when the cycle path is all bumpy, and isn't used . . . That car there [he shows us a car parked in the middle of the cycle path] is a sign of unease (president of the District Council).

However, the linkage between signs of incivility and demands for security were not apparent in La Leccia.

> There's no delinquency around here. You can't say. . . if you think. . . this is a neighbourhood where you can peacefully go for a walk, where in the summer you can have a quiet walk in the evening without any problems. You see people strolling with their grandchildren, with baby carriages (president of the District Council).

The reaction of the residents[11] was their scant participation in solution of the neighbourhood's problems, both those concerning the apartment blocks and those concerning the area's public spaces. In the apartment blocks, it was rare to find forms of self-organization, and, in the absence of administrators able to mediate with the housing agency, the time taken to deal with problems grew longer.

> With Casalp, the main door was missing because nobody ever bothered about it, including me [. . .] you'd go to Casalp once, and then a second time, and then a third. The third time, you said to yourself, 'That's it, I've had enough, I won't go any more'. Then the main door was broken [. . .] so it was removed. The gap remained for a full year. When it rained, the water came in, when it was windy, loads of leaves and litter were blown inside. There are no administrators in this building (woman, aged 36–50, resident for more than twenty years).

Nor did the residents of La Leccia participate to any significant extent in political representation bodies like the *Consiglio di Zona* (District Council). In this case, too,

[11] We carried out interviews with residents in apartment in all the three blocks of the area, collecting the points of view both of those who live in the district since its construction, both residents of the most recent, both men, both women.

the residents' scant participation was due to their disbelief that the local institutions could change anything.

> The fact is that at La Leccia it wasn't possible to elect the Consiglio di Zona with the last legislature because there were no candidates. At Scopaia they participate more because it's a new district. This district is now thirty years old and has reached the terminal stage... I mean, nothing more will be done, it can't improve (president of the District Council).

In La Leccia, the sense of isolation and abandonment was accompanied by a lack of use of public spaces. The only people who used green areas and parks were pre-adolescents and young people. The neglected public spaces became empty uninhabited spaces. Some of the residents interviewed was young mothers with little babies, who express their difficulties in living the green areas of the neighbourhood, as exemplified by the experience recounted by a mother in regard to use of the park: the empty uninhabited areas become dangerous spaces.

> They put in playground equipment, I don't know if you've seen it, all pretty and made of wood, but they didn't take care of it, and they blamed the kids for breaking it. But it wasn't true. We used to take the children, but they got splinters in their hands. I mean, it was a bit dangerous (woman, aged 36–50, resident for more than twenty years).

At Barriera Garibaldi, too, there was a perception of incivility and a sense of having been abandoned by the institutions. But the residents did not react by not using public spaces as at La Leccia. The public areas were very popular: the residents lived in the square, the building courtyards, and the streets.

Sociality at La Guglia was far from being interpretable in terms of the form assumed by spaces in the neighbourhood. Spaces that an external observer saw as 'ugly' and 'neglected' could on the contrary produce positive feelings, a sense of belonging, and even aesthetic appreciation among the residents – as in the case of the obelisk or 'the tree of the dead birds'. Nevertheless, there were also neglected spaces which the residents perceived as abandoned by the institutions and which generated a sense of insecurity. Although the "dirty and poorly lit" entry passages were used only to access the inner courtyards, the residents regarded them as dangerous. They passed through them quickly so as not to encounter "hoodies".

Unlike at La Leccia, the neglect of public spaces was blamed on several actors. The established residents felt themselves responsible for the care of places, and they attributed their sense of insecurity to outsiders. The elderly established residents mainly blamed drug addicts for episodes of petty crime which jeopardized the so-called 'block face' (Suttles 1972) – the area outside the building where children could play without supervision. "Nowadays, you can only park cars in the courtyard"; "you can't leave the doors open any more"; "there are syringes in the local park, there are too many junkies".

All the residents felt neglected by the institutions, and they accused Casalp of not maintaining the neighbourhood as it should. The established residents often reacted to this situation. Some elderly residents did not wait for the housing agency to intervene, but acted on their own: for example, by going to the park and clearing it of syringes. Shared hardship but also the intensity of relations induced some residents to interact not only as neighbours but also as a group. The person representing the residents in each building often collected complaints and acted as a spokesperson in dealings with Casalp. In some extreme situations, action took the form of outright public protest.

> Um. . .we actually went . . . from Casalp rumours . . . we were really angry because . . . rats down in the entrance, we couldn't take it any more. Walls, well, you've seen for yourself what they were like. . . in the entrance, and we were fed up. We went to get advice from [a Democratic Party politician], who said: "Guys, you have to wait, you have to wait", and we said "That's it! We can't stand it any more!" The situation had begun to be really unliveable. We came home and the protest began. We wrote on the walls, we hung banners from . . . we called the journalists, the television, and Telecentro and Italia 7 came (woman, aged 36–50, resident for fewer than twenty years).

Sense of Community and Conflicts

In La Leccia the interviews showed that there was a weak sense of solidarity and community. The area had been built quite recently, in the 1980s, and many of its inhabitants had long experience of other areas in the city. When recounting their life stories, many of the residents talked about the neighbourhoods in which they had previously lived, and where the sense of community was stronger, and about the difficulties that they had encountered when they arrived in La Leccia, where they found it more difficult to build neighbourhood ties.

> I got a bit depressed . . . It's cut off . . . where I was before there were shops, you made friends with the shopkeepers. If I wanted to go five minutes away down to San Jacopo, I'd go to a friend's shop, to the butcher's, and stay there for a chat, it was more friendly . . . (woman, aged 70, resident for ten years).

> I came back here, I said I hope I've found a big family because for me a block of flats is like a family . . . it was just like it had been in the old days in Livorno in the old quarters. When we were kids . . . if someone needed something . . . had a temperature, my mother used to say "go and wash a couple of dishes for her". It was all a family, but here I've found a lot of unpleasantness (woman, aged 51–66, resident for two years).

The difficulties of creating neighbourhood ties were reflected in the reception given to newcomers in places of formalized aggregation like the parish – as emphasised by a priest of the diocese comprising the two districts of Leccia and Scopaia.

> Here I find it extremely difficult to get people together. . . In this community it's not that. . . I saw in the parish where I was previously that if someone new came to mass, there'd be someone who went up to them. . . to say. . . welcome. Here no. . . I haven't gained this impression: if a newcomer arrives, they're ignored (priest, diocese of Leccia-Scopaia).

The difficulties of building neighbourly relations also derived from conflicts among residents. These took the form of everyday micro-conflicts or quarrels of greater intensity (in one case, a dispute was reported by the newspapers and the police investigated). As the residents recounted their life histories, they described micro-conflicts over claims not so much to 'fixed territories' – i.e. geographically delimited ones, like private courtyards and homes, the right to which is established by law – as to 'situational territories', i.e. ones claimed through their use (Goffman 1971), like benches in public areas, parks and communal spaces.

These conflicts mostly occurred between two different social groups in the neighbourhood: on the one hand, pre-adolescents and young people (and their families); on the other, neighbourhood families. They related mainly to the right to use common areas like the inner courtyards, and green spaces like the local parks. The young people and pre-adolescents hung out in those spaces, played, made a noise, and rode their motor scooters, and the other families contested their right to frequent them. The conflicts arose from claims to the use of 'situational territories' (Goffman 1971), in regard to which both groups asserted their right to determine the rules of use and to structure licit and illicit practices beyond the formal rules

> It's a long and nasty story. In a certain sense it's nasty because even though I live well here, it's unpleasant living with some people, so life is bad. They come here with their dogs and they do just as they please, these kids, they play and they do all sorts, so it's lousy here for that reason (man, aged 66–80, resident for more than twenty years).

> By law I can let my children play in the courtyard. Why do we have a courtyard if I can't take it easy on a day off at home? Why can't I let them go down to the courtyard for while because I'll get into a scrap? Because the people have come to Leccia, because it's a dormitory (woman, aged 36–50, resident for more than twenty years).

La Guglia arose from a process of urban segregation, of moving the working class out of the city centre, but the effects of segregation are not necessarily always wholly negative. The concentration of residences in the neighbourhood has meant that similar types of people live nearby, and it has been a simple matter to develop social relationships with them. Stability in the procedure for assigning flats has done the rest: it has developed traditions and sentiments that have created a sense of community and turned the residents into true neighbours – although there was also the risk that it would not do so.

The older inhabitants – the 'established' – know each other in many different roles simultaneously: as neighbours, colleagues at work, friends, and relatives. There has been a high level of endogamy in the neighbourhood: many residents have married people living in the same building, or in nearby buildings.

The forms of social relations born in the decades following the Second World War have lasted until today, even though they have obviously had to take account of the changes brought about by transformations in the neighbourhood and the arrival of new residents. It is these relationships above all that fail to survive in the same way in the new generation (Cellini and Saracino 2013).

For young people who can easily move and maintain relations at a distance with people living in other neighbourhoods of the city, the opportunity to have 'warm' interpersonal relationships is tied to a far lesser extent to physical proximity. The place of residence becomes a secondary variable, which does not prevent mobility over a broader area and activity outside the neighbourhood (Gardini and Masiello 2011). For the long-standing residents of La Guglia, it is the key space in their everyday urban lives: it contributes to define who they are and what life-opportunities they will have; it gives them access to material and social resources, and enables them to construct social and symbolic capital (Borlini 2010).

The district has a history tied to the date of its construction and to a stability of its residents connected with places and the use made of them. This history is constantly recounted by the more elderly residents and handed down from generation to generation, thus contributing to the localization of identity.[12]

In fact, however, the older residents recount an idealized version of the past. They talk of a safer type of society, of a quiet neighbourhood where residents could gather in the street, where life was good, and everyone knew everyone. Their image of the past is idealized to the point where even the deprivation and conflicts of the old days that emerge from the interviews become pleasant experiences: the Fascist era, with controls and denunciations of communists; dealing in contraband cigarettes and American products in the 1950s; immigration from the South (one of the blocks is called the "Sicilian Block").

Their image of the neighbourhood is very different today: the residents believe that it has become "like the Bronx", an expression that they use constantly.

> I'm happy I stayed in this area .... I like this neighbourhood because I was born in Shangay. La Guglia, Corea, Colline, Sorgenti, Salviano a bit less because I only see them when passing through, they're not neighbourhoods like those you can live in inside the courtyards. I like it, I was born here, I was born here and I really like the neighbourhood life, the people, the community, I like it, I like it. If they gave me a flat in Banditella, Banditella is nice, yes, but I wouldn't like it . . . It's not like it was, not at all. Before, when we were little kids, we lived with the doors and curtains open. Now you need two reinforced doors (man, aged 36–50, resident for fewer than twenty years).

What the residents feel is a sense of insecurity related to what in the literature is called the 'fear of crime'; a fear which concerns the safety of both persons and property (D'Aloisio 2011, 186). The crime episodes that occur are amplified, generalized, and recounted over and over again. To an external observer, however, despite its problems, the neighbourhood still seems very peaceful. For example, there is almost nobody on the streets in the evening: the 'established' accuse the 'outsiders', but both have the same daily routines and frequent the same places.

In our opinion, it is possible to identify a deeper reason for the sense of insecurity felt by the older residents. Their identities are plotted within clear spatial and symbolic coordinates. In a context where there has been no social turnover for many years (Negri and Olagnero 2001, 231), the presence of new inhabitants generates a sense of loss associated with the control of spaces and relations, with the difficulty of recognizing and being recognized. According to Wallman (1998), in fact, recognizing and being recognized creates a sense of belonging in the inhabitants of an area. At La Guglia, the sense of community constructed over the years still persists, but it is undermined by the outsiders, who disobey the shared informal rules, and have lifestyles different from those of the established residents.

[12] Places are so important for the identities of the established residents that every public space and every courtyard is identified by them with a nickname.

There are few foreign residents in La Guglia, and they have only a very limited influence on consolidated relationships; but their image among the established residents is replete with prejudices and based on stereotypes. The provision of homes to foreigners by the City of Livorno Housing Department, in particular, is viewed as an usurpation of the residents' rights.

It is mostly the multi-problem families and the drug addicts that have a destabilizing effect on the community because they do not abide by the social rules that it has laid down. The established residents are judgmental and speak ill of the multi-problem families because their members often come from unstable emotional backgrounds, because they are single-parent families, because they have many more children than the average, because they live by the day and have no stable income, because they sometimes do not pay their rent even though it is low, and because they are assisted by the social services.

The established residents and the addicts engage in an open and almost constant conflict, sometimes reported by the local newspaper. The established see the 'junkies' as only a cause of problems in the neighbourhood. Because of their precariousness in life and residence, the drug addicts see the established as privileged because they have homes and enough money to live on.

At La Guglia the difference between the two macro-types of resident identified above derives from their diverse socio-economic circumstances. But it acquires importance through the construction of social representations. The established residents use the difference as the basis for the creation of a stigma which is both a feature of exclusion and a reason for it. The emphasising of difference is a means to construct identity and a political resource for definition of the situation and collective action (Colombo 2007, 24–27). The strong bonds among the residents mean that conflicts centre on identity and membership the community, not on the usual micro-problems of life in an apartment block. Although these are present in the accounts of the inhabitants of La Guglia, they are less significant than at La Leccia, where relations among the residents are very poor.

Conclusions

Housing quality is a complex concept with several layers of meaning. The analysis of data produced from official sources or collected by means of survey forms or questionnaires does not reveal all the dimensions and sub-dimensions of housing quality. It does not consider the meanings that the actors give to such dimensions, and it may fail to grasp the interconnections among different dimensions. The ethnographic method enabled the research group to explore the complexity of the concept of housing quality in various ways, and to articulate its dimensions more efficaciously.

In our research, thanks to data furnished mainly by Casalp and the Municipality of Livorno, we obtained information relative to the legal dimension, the structural characteristics of dwellings and buildings, and the socio-economic characteristics of the residents. For example, we recorded the number of dwellings assigned under housing emergency procedures, the average rent, the year of construction and state of repair of buildings, the floor space of dwellings in square metres, the presence of disabled persons, and the type of household. These data brought out several differences between the two neighbourhoods. At Barriera Garibaldi there were numerous small flats and a high level of housing emergency. The state of maintenance of buildings was more unsatisfactory than at La Leccia, and the socio-economic circumstances of families were more problematic. But upon immersion, some of these differences attenuated. On observing the buildings, entering the flats, and interviewing the inhabitants, we found that also at La Leccia the quality of accommodation and its state of maintenance were sub-standard. Although the average rent was higher than in other SHEs in Livorno, at La Leccia there were numerous families which relied on support from local voluntary associations because of their economic difficulties.

The ethnographic research gave depth to the data and enriched them with the meanings that the actors attributed to the situations reported by the sources. By going into the field, we experienced the everyday difficulties of La Leccia families, which for instance, because of rainwater infiltration, could not use some rooms of their flats and were forced to live in less space than that assigned to them. We listened to the story recounted by Luca, who at Barriera Garibaldi was forced to sleep in a camper van parked in the courtyard because his flat was on the fourth floor without a lift and he could not climb the stairs.

As we observed in the neighbourhood and its residents we noted that some aspects of housing – relations among the residents and the relations between these and the institutions – were crucial for understanding life in the district. Whether tenants felt themselves to be the residents or only the users of their flats, their perception of the institutions and bureaucracy, their types of relations and ties – strong or weak – and their possession of a shared history, were aspects important for analysis of housing quality in a neighbourhood.

Finally, research in the field showed that the complexity of certain processes prevented separation among the dimensions of housing quality. These proved to be closely bound up with each other in everyday life. For example, the residents' perceptions of incivilities in public places and the poor quality of the neighbourhood's urban life were due to their relationships with the institutions and their sense of abandonment by the public housing agency and the local authorities. Social practices in public spaces were interconnected with relations among residents, and their sense of community and local belonging.

At La Leccia the personal stories of the inhabitants included other neighbourhoods, and resident identity was fragmented. There was a lack of symbolic places, and a powerful presence of incivilities. There was a perception of distance from the institutions among the residents, and a feeling that they had been abandoned by them. Social relations were fragile, the sense of community was weak, and there were micro-conflicts among young people, pre-adolescents, and adults.

At La Guglia personal stories reflected the history of the neighbourhood: being a resident of the neighbourhood was a significant part of personal identity; identity as a resident was continuous, and a strong sense of belonging to the neighbourhood had developed. Certain places had powerful symbolic value, social relations were strong; and there were conflicts between the established residents and outsiders.

The inhabitants of La Leccia would quarrel over a football kicked too far, or over a bench in the courtyard. Those of La Guglia aggressively preserved their identity against persons regarded as 'foreign bodies'. The residents of La Leccia had only one way to react to their poor housing conditions: that of making individual complaints to Casalp. The inhabitants of Barriera Garibaldi, thanks to their dense relations, also reacted collectively through organized protest action.

Acknowledgments The research reported in this paper was part of the "PONEC (*Public housing is not a concept*)" project funded by the Region of Tuscany ("*decreto dirigenziale*" no. 7039 of 24 December 2009). The partners in the project are the *Centro Interdisciplinare di Metodologia delle Scienze Sociali* of the University of Florence, the Livorno City Council, and Casalp S.p.A. Fondazione Michelucci provides consultancy services. The authors wish to thank the members of the research group and those persons who helped them in the field, the residents, the workers at the *Portineria sociale di condominio di Livorno*, and all those who gave them first-hand information.

References

Agenzia del Territorio. (2011). *Statistiche catastali 2010 (Catasto edilizio urbano)*. http://www.agenziaterritorio.it/sites/territorio/files/osservatorio/Tabelle%20statistiche/Statistiche_Catastali_2010.pdf. Accessed 16 Aug 2012.

Atkinson, R. (1998). *The life story interview*. London: Sage.

Atkinson, T., Cantillon, B., Marlier, E., & Nolan, B. (2002). *Social indicators – The EU and social inclusion*. Oxford: Oxford University Press.

Augé, M. (1992). *Non-lieux*. Paris: Seuil.

Authier, J. Y., Bacqué, M. H., & Guérin-Pace, F. (2007). *Le quartier. Enjeux scientifiques, actions politiques et pratiques sociale*. Paris: La Découverte.

Bagnasco, A. (1999). *Fatti sociali formati nello spazio. Cinque lezioni di sociologia urbana e regionale*. Milano: Franco Angeli.

Bichi, R. (2007). *La conduzione delle interviste nella ricerca sociale*. Roma: Carocci.

Borlini, B. (2010). Il quartiere nella città contemporanea. Come e perché occuparsene. *Quaderni di Sociologia, LIV*(52), 13–30.

Bortolotti, L. (1967). Storia dell'edilizia popolare di Livorno. *Casabella: rivista internazionale di architettura e urbanistica, 320*, 16–23.

Cellamare, C. (2011). Pratiche dell'abitare. La ricerca urbanistica e la "città degli uomini". *Etnografia e ricerca qualitativa, IV*(2), 305–316.

Cellini, E. (2008). *L'osservazione nelle scienze umane*. Milano: Franco Angeli.

Cellini, E., & Saracino, B. (2013). Re(l)azioni popolari: etnografia in un quartiere di edilizia residenziale pubblica. *Etnografia e Ricerca Qualitativa, VI*(2), 259–281.

Chiesi, L. (2004). Le inciviltà. Degrado urbano e insicurezza. In R. Selmini (Ed.), *La sicurezza urbana* (pp. 129–140). Bologna: Il Mulino.

Colombo, E. (2007). Multiculturalismo quotidiano: la differenza come vincolo e come risorsa. In E. Colombo & G. Semi (Eds.), *Multiculturalismo quotidiano. Le pratiche della differenza* (pp. 15–36). Milano: Franco Angeli.

Colombo, E., & Navarini, G. (1999). *Confini dentro la città. Antropologia della stazione centrale di Milano*. Milano: Guerini e Associati.

D'Alosio, F. (2011). Localizzare la sicurezza globale. Le molteplici dimensioni della sicurezza urbana in un quartiere napoletano. In M. Bressan & S. Tosi Cambini (Eds.), *Zone di transizione. Etnografia urbana nei quartieri e nello spazio pubblico* (pp. 167–201). Bologna: Il Mulino.

De Certeau, M. (1990). *L'invention du quotidien*. Paris: Gallimard.

Douglas, J. D. (1976). *Investigative social research: Individual and team field research*. Thousand Oaks: Sage.

Elias, N., & Scotson, J. L. (1994). *The established and the outsiders*. London: Sage.

EuroFound. (2006). *First European Quality of Life Survey: Social dimensions of housing*. Luxembourg: Office for Official Publications of the European Communities.

Eurostat. (2010). *Income and living conditions in Europe*. Luxembourg: Publications Office of the European Union.

Fischer, C. (1982). *To dwell among friends: Personal networks in town and city*. Chicago: University of Chicago Press.

Foucault, M. (2001). *Spazi altri. I luoghi delle eterotopie*. Milano: Mimesis.

Gardini, E., & Masiello, S. (Eds.). (2011). *Periferia. Sguardi sociologici*. Roma: Nuova cultura.

Gasparini, A. (2000). *La sociologia degli spazi. Luoghi, città, società*. Roma: Carocci.

Genestier, P. (1999). Le sortilège du quartier: quand le lieu est censé faire lien. *Les Annales de la recherche urbaine, 82*, 142–153.

Glaser, B. G., & Strauss, A. L. (1967). *The discovery of grounded theory: Strategies for qualitative research*. Chicago: Aldine Publishing Company.

Gobo, G. (2001). *Descrivere il mondo. Teoria e pratica del metodo etnografico in sociologia*. Roma: Carocci.

Goffman, E. (1971). *Relations in pubblic*. New York: Basic Book.

Goffman, E. (1974). *Frame analysis. An essay on the organization of experience*. New York: Harper & Row.

Halbwachs, M. (1968). *La mémoire collective*. Paris: Press Universitaires de France.

La Cecla, F. (2005). *Perdersi. L'uomo senza ambiente*. Roma-Bari: Laterza.

Lynch, K. (1960). *The image of the city*. Cambridge: MIT Press.

Mela, A. (1999). *Sociologia delle città*. Milano: Franco Angeli.

Negri, N., & Olagnero, M. (2001). Poveri e non poveri: i confini incerti dell'utenza di edilizia pubblica a Torino. In M. L. Bianco (Ed.), *L'Italia delle diseguaglianze* (pp. 227–267). Roma: Carocci.

Negri, N., & Saraceno, C. (2000). Povertà, disoccupazione ed esclusione sociale. *Stato e Mercato, 59*, 175–210.

Olagnero, M. (1998). I muri e le barriere. Il disagio abitativo tra crisi del welfare, crisi del mercato e trasformazioni della famiglia. *Rassegna Italiana di Sociologia, XXXIX*(1), 43.

Pierini, R. (2001). 100 anni di case popolari a Livorno. In R. Pierini (Ed.), *La città distante. Piani e progetti di edilizia residenziale pubblica* (pp. 185–226). Pisa: Edizioni ETS.

Poggio, T. (2009). Le principali dimensioni della disuguaglianza abitativa in Italia. In A. Brandolini, C. Saraceno, & A. Schizzerotto (Eds.), *Dimensioni della disuguaglianza in Italia: Povertà, salute, abitazione* (pp. 273–292). Bologna: Il Mulino.

Regione Toscana. (2012). *Abitare in Toscana – Anno 2012. Primo rapporto sulla condizione abitativa*. Osservatorio Sociale Regionale. http://toscana-notizie.it/wp-content/uploads/2012/04/Rapporto-condizione-abitativa-2012.pdf. Accessed 16 Aug 2012.

Ricci, R. (Ed.). (1997). *Povertà abitativa in Italia, 1989–1993*. Roma: Commissione sulla povertà e l'esclusione sociale in Italia.

Sacchetti, F. (2012). Creatività e Categorie tra quantitativo e qualitativo. In C. Cipolla, A. De Lillo, & E. Ruspini (Eds.), *Il sociologo, le sirene e le pratiche di integrazione* (pp. 255–272). Milano: Franco Angeli.

Salzman, P. C. (1989). The failure of solitary fieldwork. *Anthropology Newsletter, 30*(4), 26–28.

Sclavi, M., et al. (2002). *Avventure urbane. Progettare la città con gli abitanti*. Milano: Elèuthera.
Sen, A. (1985). *Commodities and capabilities*. Amsterdam: North Holland.
Simmel, G. (1908). *Soziologie. Untersuchungen über die Formen der Vergesellschaftung*. Berlin: Duncker & Humblot.
Suttles, G. (1972). *The social construction of communities*. Chicago: University of Chicago Press.
Tosi, A. (Ed.). (1994). *La casa: il rischio e l'esclusione. Rapporto IRS sul disagio abitativo in Italia*. Milano: Franco Angeli.
Trigilia, C. (1983). Sub-cultura rossa e partito comunista. In S. Belligni (Ed.), *La giraffa e il liocorno. Il PCI dagli anni '70 al nuovo decennio* (pp. 142–150). Milano: Franco Angeli.
Wallman, S. (1998). New identities and local factors – Or when is home in town a good move? In N. Rapport & A. Dawson (Eds.), *Migrants of identity. Perceptions of home in a world of movement* (pp. 181–205). London: Berg.
Zajczyk, F., Borlini, B., Memo, F., & Mugnano, S. (2005). *Milano. Quartieri periferici tra incertezza e trasformazione*. Milano: Bruno Mondadori.

Chapter 4
Making the Ordinary Extraordinary: A Fresh Look at Satisfaction in Communities

Craig A. Talmage

What Is It About Communities? Important Pieces of the Puzzle

> The biggest threat to any individual or society is the loss of hope, hopelessness. . .The key is to believe, to believe we can make things better.—Paul Johnson, Former Mayor of the City of Phoenix (1990–1994).

This paper seeks to account the role of individual satisfaction in enriching community development. Satisfaction is an affective feeling people experience and can describe. It is an act of judgment; an individual makes a rational decision about their level of satisfaction (Mannell and Kleiber 1997; Herzberg 1966, 1987). People are motivated to attain satisfaction, specifically to satisfy their needs (Mannell and Kleiber 1997; Maslow 1954; Herzberg 1966). Satisfaction has permeated into and prevailed in different research fields including but not limited to product development, organizational development, and community development. Using satisfaction from multiple research fields, this paper proposes a new model for manipulating satisfaction to enrich events, associations, and communities.

Researchers and practitioners in the business sector continue to debate the best approaches to motivate employees, while the community sector has continued to debate the best ways to motivate community members. Rarely have these debates comingled in the literature. The business sector has worked to influence employee satisfaction to increase engagement and productivity, whereas the community sector has approached its desire to increase engagement not only through policy formation but by influencing community members' attitudes (Bellah et al. 1985). Thus, research yields many explanations for community satisfaction and its

C.A. Talmage (✉)
School of Community Resources and Development, Arizona State University, 411 N. Central Ave. Suite 550, Phoenix, AZ 85004-0685, USA
e-mail: ctalmage@asu.edu

F. Maggino (ed.), *A New Research Agenda for Improvements in Quality of Life*, Social Indicators Research Series 57, DOI 10.1007/978-3-319-15904-1_4

outcomes, but the community sector may have more to learn from the business sector when working to improve community satisfaction and its outcomes.

This paper identifies the specific aspects of communities, associations, and events that influence satisfaction to develop new research questions, models, and interventions to better communities. The main philosophical question asked is, "What do people want from their communities?" Organizational theorists like Herzberg et al. (1959) asked a similar question; they asked, "What do people want from their jobs?" (p. 107). These questions provide a point for comparison regarding attitudes and motivation in both workplaces and communities. Thus, lessons to be learned can be found in both venues through understanding satisfaction.

Revisiting Satisfaction as Two-Factors

This paper proposes a revisit to Frederick Herzberg's Two-Factor Theory also known as the Motivation to Work Theory (Herzberg 1966). Over 50 years ago, Herzberg and colleagues (1959) found that satisfaction and dissatisfaction were distinctly different in nature and influenced by different job factors. Prior to 1957, many studies saw satisfaction simply as a dichotomous affective state. One was either satisfied or dissatisfied (Herzberg et al. 1957). If both satisfaction and dissatisfaction result from different outcomes in organizational settings, then can the same findings be observed in community settings?

As mentioned earlier, the central philosophical question that Herzberg built his work upon was "what do people want from their jobs" (Herzberg et al. 1959, p. 107). Herzberg and colleagues (1959) in line with humanists like Abraham Maslow (1954) believed individuals had the right to determine what was best for their lives; they had the right to determine what satisfies them. Herzberg and colleagues (1959) utilized a critical incidents approach to identify factors that contributed to satisfaction and dissatisfaction.

The critical incidents helped identify exceptionally high or low moments in the experiences of different persons. The incidents were recorded and subjected to content analysis because of their highly qualitative nature (Herzberg et al. 1959). In 1959, the motivator and hygiene factors were identified, and in 1966, Herzberg's dual continuum appeared (see Fig. 4.1) positing job satisfaction and job dissatisfaction as two distinct factors (Herzberg 1966). The idea of two different continua was a paradigmatic shift in the management field because separating these two factors into two unipolar continuums departed from previous conceptualizations of satisfaction-dissatisfaction as a bipolar continuum with a singular zero point (Herzberg 1966; Bassett-Jones and Lloyd 2005).

The satisfaction continuum deals with seeking growth from job tasks and is influenced by motivators (Herzberg et al. 1959; Herzberg 1966). Looking at the figure, one can see that satisfaction derived from the motivators leads to job satisfaction, but the absence of the motivators is not dissatisfaction but no job satisfaction (Herzberg 1966). No job satisfaction is most easily conceptualized as boredom (Herzberg 1966).

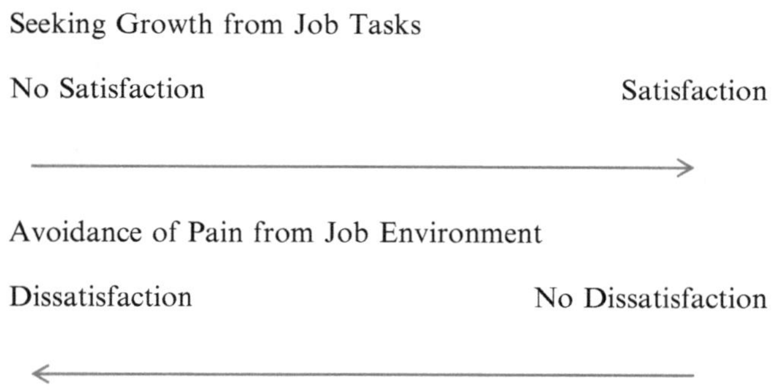

Fig. 4.1 Job satisfaction and dissatisfaction continua

Dissatisfaction fell on a different continuum dealing with concerns to avoid pain from one's environments. Dissatisfaction is influenced by hygiene (Herzberg et al. 1959; Herzberg 1966). Dissatisfaction derived from hygiene leads to job dissatisfaction, but contentment with these factors is not satisfaction but no job dissatisfaction (Herzberg 1966). No job satisfaction is described as temporary satisfaction or short-term positive affect (Herzberg 1966).

The goal of Herzberg's job enrichment was to maximize satisfaction and minimize dissatisfaction (Herzberg 1966, 1968, 1987). Consistently, the service quality literature continues to stress this point emphasizing the maximization of satisfaction and minimization of dissatisfaction (Dawes and Rowley 1999). Satisfaction and dissatisfaction are not opposites but separate concepts (Bleuel 1990; Johnston 1995; Herzberg 1966, 1974, 1987; Scitovsky 1976; Carvalho et al. 2010). Satisfaction does not necessarily emerge when dissatisfaction is removed, and dissatisfaction may have a stronger and longer lasting effect on behavior than satisfaction (Bleuel 1990; Johnston 1995; Findlay 1967).

Table 4.1 outlines hygiene and motivators, two qualitatively distinct factors. Hygiene has been described as being more related to the job context and influences job dissatisfaction (Crompton 2003). The motivators appear to be more related to the job content and influence job satisfaction (Crompton 2003). Hygiene is more extrinsic in nature; while, the motivators are more intrinsic in nature (Crompton 2003; Oliver 1997). Hygiene needs to be sufficient for a worker to have the potential to be motivated to be more productive; however, motivators spur long-term productivity and engagement (Herzberg 1966).

The absence of motivators may drive persons to become what Herzberg (1966) called hygiene seekers. These persons, because they lack opportunities for psychological growth, are driven to obtain the temporary satisfaction that hygiene offers (Herzberg 1966). These persons are not only victims of their environment but also become possibly neurotic, because they must react in order to psychologically cope with their situations (Herzberg 1966). Hygiene essentially acts like heroine taking more and more each time to be satisfactory (Herzberg 1966).

Table 4.1 Hygiene and motivators

Hygiene	Motivator
Company policy and administration[a]	Achievement[a]
Supervision[a]	Recognition[a]
Interpersonal relations[a]	Work itself[a]
Working conditions[a]	Responsibility[a]
Salary[a,b]	Advancement[a]
Status[b]	Possibility of growth[b]
Job security[b]	
Effects on personal life[b]	

Adapted from Herzberg (1966)
[a]Denotes first-level job factor
[b]Denotes second-level job-attitude factor

On the contrary, motivator seekers are seen to have a greater degree of overall mental health by Herzberg (1966). Motivator seekers search for opportunities for learning and psychological growth. They place greater importance on higher order needs (i.e. belonging or actualization) compared to hygiene seekers who place greater importance on lower order needs (i.e. money for security) (Herzberg 1966; Sutaria 1980).

After the publication of Herzberg's (1966) seminal work on Two-Factor Theory, a debate erupted among researchers in the management field, and the debate became ugly (Bockman 1971). Some felt that the two-factor concept could easily be arbitrarily constructed and imposed on situations, and it was not derived from reliable nor valid aggregate data (Bockman 1971). It is also likely that those working to debunk Herzberg's (1968, 1987) theory likely misunderstood its intricacies (Bockman 1971).

Additionally, it has been argued that the theory neglects to assess the interaction effects of hygiene and motivators (Bockman 1971); however, Herzberg and colleagues' (1959) foundational study found that motivators do not exclusively lead to satisfaction, and hygiene does not exclusively lead to dissatisfaction. Thus, dissatisfaction with motivators may be related to decreases in engagement or the absence of engagement (termed boredom), and satisfaction from hygiene may be related to increases in engagement (termed movement) though the effect is not likely long lasting (see Herzberg et al. 1959; Herzberg 1966; Sachau 2007).

Many of Herzberg's contemporaries have agreed that he was wrong about interpersonal relationships, such as relationships with bosses, coworkers, and subordinates (Sachau 2007). While Herzberg believed that relationships only served to move persons to action, others like Sachau (2007), a former student of Herzberg, believe that certain interpersonal relationships can lead to psychological growth and development. Sachau (2007) cites that family relationships and friendships can lead to either psychological growth or pain avoidance. Finally, Wagner and Harter (2006) and Csikzentmihalyi (1997) have linked engagement to friendships at work.

However, it is no wonder why others to this day still defend Herzberg's approach (e.g., Sachau 2007; Belias and Koustelios 2014). It appears useful in so far that it can still provide some insight or explanation for our own actions which are influenced by our perceptions (e.g, Smith and Miller 1978; White 1980). Looking at Table 4.2 (soon to be discussed) and the examples to be discussed, there appears to be differences consistent with Herzberg's work, but very few have linked his theory to community settings.

The Factors That Contribute to Satisfaction and Dissatisfaction in Communities

Table 4.2 shows many of the community factors identified as contributors to community satisfaction and dissatisfaction in the literature. These factors contributing to satisfaction and dissatisfaction are drawn primarily from research on

Table 4.2 Previous contributing factors to community satisfaction

Factor	Publications
Physical environment	Allen et al. (1991)
Urban activity & noise	Amérigo and Aragonés (1990) and Zehner (1971)
Open spaces, natural resources	Amérigo and Aragonés (1990), Fried (1982), Kaplan (1984), (2001), Medalia (1964), and Zehner (1971)
Infrastructure	Amérigo and Aragonés (1990) and Zehner (1971)
Formal education	Allen et al. (1991)
Educational service	Orthner et al. (1990) and Sirgy et al. (2000)
Thermal insulation	Amérigo and Aragonés (1988)
Medical services	Allen et al. (1991) and Orthner et al. (1990)
Municipal & public services	Allen et al. (1991), Fried (1982), Orthner et al. (1990), and Sirgy et al. (2000)
Transportation & accessibility	Zehner (1971)
Safety & privacy	Amérigo and Aragonés (1988), (1990), and Fried (1982)
Crime	Miller et al. (1980)
Government	Orthner et al. (1990)
Economy	Allen et al. (1991), Brown (1993), Filkins et al. (2000), Orthner et al. (1990), Rodgers (1980), and Sirgy et al. (2000)
Standard of living	Rodgers (1980)
Taxes	Rodgers (1980) and Sirgy et al. (2000)
Status	Fried (1982)
Socioeconomic status	Sampson (1991)
Recreation & leisure	Allen et al. (1991), Payne and Schaumleffel (2008), Molnar et al. (1979), Fuiguit and Zuiches (1975), Orthner et al. (1990), Vreugdenhil and Rigby (1987), and Zehner (1971)
Social support, bonds, & participation	Buttel et al. (1979), Hughey and Bardo (1984), Orthner et al. (1990), Speare (1974), and Ikeda et al. (2008)
Arts, aesthetics, & culture	White (1985) and Grillo et al. (2010)

communities of place; though, parallels can be seen in other fields such as communities of interest. Both physical and social environmental factors significantly influence (dis)satisfaction (e.g., Zehner 1971; Goudy 1977).

The community satisfaction (and dissatisfaction) literature has revealed that both a community's physical environment and infrastructure are important to (dis) satisfaction (e.g, Allen et al. 1991; Amérigo and Aragonés 1990; Zehner 1971). Kaplan (1984, 2001) has linked opportunities to appreciate and proximity to the natural outdoor environment to residential engagement and other psychological benefits. Medalia (1964) noted that air pollution in cities was linked to community dissatisfaction. Finally, Campbell et al. (1976) found that educational institutions, roads, recreation facilities, and police protection related to community (dis) satisfaction.

Orthner et al. (1990) have suggested that community services do not significantly impact satisfaction unless they are of poor quality or are absent. Furthermore, these services are necessary but not sufficient to increase community satisfaction; thus, responding to community needs is more effective than improving the actual quality of community services (Orthner et al. 1990; Brackertz and Kenley 2002). Similarly, Herzberg and colleagues (1959) found that poor environmental conditions of workplaces and perceptions of top management and administration of resources were contributors to job dissatisfaction.

Safety and privacy have also been consistently linked to community (dis)satisfaction (Amérigo and Aragonés 1988, 1990; Fried 1982). For example, Miller and colleagues (1980) found fear of crime to be their most salient factor of influence on neighborhood satisfaction. Policing and evaluations of police and government involvement in the community influence satisfaction (Pennell 1978). Again, Herzberg and colleagues (1959) found that environmental conditions, specifically safety and interpersonal relationships, were related to dissatisfaction.

Researchers have shown that governance and economic factors are related to community (dis)satisfaction (Allen et al. 1991; Brown 1993; Filkins et al. 2000; Orthner et al. 1990; Rodgers 1980; Sirgy et al. 2000), specifically income, employment, and taxes. For instance, Rodgers (1980) has shown that in residential settings the standard of living, evaluations of local taxes, and satisfaction with finances were positively related to satisfaction and were also strong drivers of dissatisfaction. Herzberg and colleagues (1959) also found that perceptions of top management and administration of resources were contributors to dissatisfaction.

Socioeconomic status has also been linked to satisfaction and dissatisfaction (Fried 1982; Sampson 1991). For instance, persons of lower socioeconomic status often show lower levels of civic engagement likely related to community satisfaction (Costa and Kahn 2004). Knack and Keefer (2003) have even suggested that persons only become civically engaged if they have something to gain. Consistently, Herzberg and colleagues (1959) found that a person's perception of his or her status in an organization was related to job dissatisfaction; however, advancement was related to job satisfaction.

Recreation and leisure also influences community (dis)satisfaction (Allen et al. 1991; Fuiguit and Zuiches 1975; Orthner et al. 1990; Payne and Schaumleffel

2008). In fact, Molnar and colleagues (1979) have found that the amount and quality of recreation and leisure opportunities in a community were negatively related to dissatisfaction. Additionally, Vreugdenhil and Rigby (1987) found recreational facilities to be an important factor in explaining satisfaction.

Grillo and colleagues (2010) and White (1985) linked cultural and social factors to community (dis)satisfaction. The social factors of communities that contribute to satisfaction include informal social support (Orthner et al. 1990; White 1985), social bonds (Speare 1974), and social interaction (Campbell et al. 1976; Fried 1982). More recently, Csikzentmihalyi (1997) has suggested that the most positive experiences in persons' lives are those experienced with friends. Finally, Herzberg and colleagues (1959) found that interpersonal relationships and supervision to be related to job dissatisfaction; however, Herzberg's contemporaries (see Sachau 2007) have noted that interpersonal relationships may also be drivers of job satisfaction.

The community factors just described fall in line with Herzberg and colleagues' (1959) ordering of factors (see Table 4.1 for reference): first-level factors (see Herzberg 1966), objective aspects of the community environment related to satisfaction and its outcomes (i.e. crime); and second-level factors, perceptions of or attitudes linked to specific aspects of the community environment (i.e. fear of crime). These two factors make up what Herzberg and colleagues (1959) referred to as the factors-attitudes-effects complex, whereas effects are not only influenced by first- and second-level factors but affect these factors as well. The factors-attitudes-effects complex was largely derived from Kurt Lewin's (1931) position that all behavior is a function of the interaction between a person and his or her environment.

Unfortunately, research endeavors that have focused on community (dis)satisfaction appear to have honed in more heavily on factors that contribute to dissatisfaction than satisfaction. These factors appear to be outside of an individual's locus of control. Thus, more research is needed on those factors that contribute to community satisfaction. These factors encompass community members' evaluations of their personal role in their communities and how they have bettered their own lives and the lives of others. These factors likely parallel Herzberg's (1966) motivators and can be incorporated into communities, associations, and events. This line of research is important since community researchers like Block and Zautra (1981) have found that life satisfaction is influenced by motivators and psychological distress is influenced by hygiene.

Connecting Community Satisfaction and Dissatisfaction with Community Outcomes

Much of the literature already reviewed has described residential and neighborhood settings, but other forms of communities such as professional associations, faith communities, community organizations, or student groups may benefit from answering these questions (e.g., Amérigo and Aragonés 1988, 1990; Fried 1982; Zehner 1971). A sole focus on communities from a systematic and macro-lens has the potential disadvantage of overlooking the reasons individuals choose to be active, involved, or engaged in a community and bring about community change. This research, through providing a summary of satisfaction on a macro-scale, posits similar themes on more meso- and micro-scales like neighborhoods or associations.

Though many of our real motives for behavior may be unconscious to us (Iso-Ahola 1980); satisfaction and dissatisfaction, which we are conscious of, have important effects. Researchers have well-documented the negative outcomes of dissatisfaction. These effects include leaving a community, community instability, and a lower quality of life (Bach and Smith 1977; Filkins et al. 2000; Heaton et al. 1979). For example, dissatisfaction has been linked to the decision to leave a community, while satisfaction has been linked to the decision to stay (Rossi 1955; Schulze et al. 1963).

Community (dis)satisfaction has often been connected to civic engagement (e.g., Allen et al. 1991). Civic engagement can take many forms such as volunteerism and associational involvement; yet, many of these actions have been shown to be more reactionary to combat community deficiencies or problems as opposed to proactive actions that lead to overall community betterment (e.g., Knack and Keefer 2003). Grillo and colleagues (2010) discussed whether disengaged populations required a different approach than populations that are not yet engaged; however, the differences between disengaged and not yet engaged were not clearly defined (Grillo et al. 2010). Not yet engaged populations appear to need more social offerings, while disengaged populations appear to need more public offerings (Grillo et al. 2010). Social offerings were operationalized as opportunities to meet and interact with people, and public offerings were those that met the basic needs of the community. Thus, contentment with one's basic needs may lead to apathy, such that civic engagement decreases when problems dissipate consistent with Herzberg's (1966) Two-Factor Theory.

Another question arises, "Is there a difference between civic engagement and civic disengagement," both macro-level concepts. "Civic engagement refers to the ways in which citizens participate in the life of a community in order to improve conditions for others or to help shape the community's future" (Adler and Goggin 2005, p. 236). Civic engagement falls on a continuum spanning from informal private actions to formal collective actions (Adler and Goggin 2005).

Civic disengagement is absent from many continuums and models. Using logic one could conclude that the outcomes of engagement and disengagement should oppose each other. If the outcome of engagement is active involvement, then is the outcome of disengagement no involvement? Putnam (2000) defines civic disengagement as an unraveling of civic engagement and social capital in American society; but, perhaps the outcomes of disengagement are far different or worse than previously thought—such as migration or sabotage. The motives that bring out the best in people may be the same motives that bring out the worst in people (Mannell and Kleiber 1997). These types of questions characterize the common differences between one- and two-factor theories of satisfaction. These types of questions permeate further into the subcomponents of community systems such associations and events; however, these deep-reaching questions have been easily overlooked in research regarding these subcomponents.

Association Satisfaction: An Overlooked Community Factor

> It's interesting to talk macro-, but what if we took a breath and thought micro-, thought about me, my world, my streets?—Billy Thrall, CityServe Arizona.

The same types of questions have permeated into research on involvement in associations. The differences between passive support and active involvement have been debated often regarding engagement in associations. The dichotomization of these as two distinct constructs may actually hinder organizations that are looking to move persons from being passively supportive to actively involved. Thus, there still appears to be merit for more theoretical development regarding association satisfaction including Herzberg's (1966) Two-Factor Theory.

Aside from corporations, associations are likely the most powerful organized groups in the United States. McKnight (2013) writes, in reference of de Tocqueville, of the historical importance and power of associations, "they (associations and their members) were taking power by making power through community action" (p. 3). Each person within and event held by an association has the potential to uniquely generate social capacity (McKnight 1987, 2013).

Engagement outside of the private sector has been posited to be declining (Putnam 1995). Engagement can be described as a person's sense of affiliation or identification with an association (Albert and Dignam 2010; Dalton and Dignam 2007). Affiliation fosters a notion of shared identity (Dalton and Dignam 2007). Dalton and Dignam (2007) write, "When people affiliate, they let the world around them know that they share an important quality with this group" (p. 19). Affiliation is the precursor to involvement; thus, it is important to understand why persons choose to affiliate or to no longer affiliate (Dalton and Dignam 2007).

Motives for joining an association are related to individual levels of participation (Wollebaek and Selle 2003). Involvement is dependent on material motives (tangible benefits), purposive motives (altruistic ideals), and solidary benefits (social interactions and status) (Holmes and Slater 2012; Caldwell and Andereck 1994; King and Walker 1992). Passive members appear to be more focused on material motives than purposive motives and solidary benefits (Slater 2003). Holmes and Slater (2012) posited that active members are more motivated by purposive motives and solidary benefits; however, the relationship remains unconfirmed.

Formal affiliation often begins with the paying of a membership or an event fee. The next natural step for an affiliating person might be to give to an association. Gifts of time and money have been shown to be both altruistic and self-serving (Gazley and Dignam 2010). Members may give to improve society but also to receive the indirect benefits (i.e., satisfaction) they expect from the associations to which they contribute (Gazley and Dignam 2010). Thus, a difference between intrinsic and extrinsic motivation appears (see Deci and Ryan 1985). Givers appear to be much more intrinsically motivated, than extrinsically motivated. Consistent with Herzberg's (1966, 1974, 1987) work, factors that provide members with a sense of achievement or responsibility and are focused on the work of the association are seen as more important than extrinsic rewards such as increasing one's status in an association.

Dalton and Dignam (2007) studied association members' decisions to join and affiliate or to drop affiliation with an association. They contend that members affiliate based on their value perceptions regarding benefits of affiliation. Those whose involvement appeared to be more serious or to show greater commitment or involvement showed higher perceptions of value regarding associations (Dalton and Dignam 2007). Those who were more involved rated associations more favorably, believed there will be a greater need for associations in the future, and were more likely to promote and recommend an association to friends or colleagues (Dalton and Dignam 2007). Another benefit of affiliation is building social capital, such that persons who are affiliated with more associations are more likely to show higher levels of social capital and its subcomponents: Trust, social networks, and civic engagement (Wollebaek and Selle 2002).

Despite the amount of research on involvement and engagement in associations, there is much less on the satisfaction of association members and how those associations influence their larger communities. The reasons for members to give to and become and remain involved in associations appear to be due to the intrinsic benefits they receive from the association (Gazley and Dignam 2008, 2010). For instance, recognition and interpersonal relationships are important for involvement. Gazley and Dignam (2008) wrote about the "power of the direct ask" (p. 3). Members were more likely to participate in associations if they were simply asked.

Members appear to cease giving and become less involved or leave associations because of extrinsic factors (Gazley and Dignam 2010). For example, Gazley and Dignam (2008) found that "family, work, and geography can all limit volunteer participation" (p. 3). They noted that their study participants realized that most of the reasons people volunteer for professional associations are under an association's control. Thus, Herzberg's (1966, 1987) Two-Factor Theory and work on intrinsic and extrinsic motivation (Deci and Ryan 1985) can be linked to satisfaction in associations as well.

Association satisfaction and dissatisfaction warrants, nay deserves, further study because "groups are the crucible in which civil society is created" (Fine and Harrington 2004, p. 344). Satisfaction as opposed to obligation is what keeps volunteers involved, active, and engaged members of associations and citizens of their communities. Putnam (2000) argued, "What really matters from the point of view of social capital and civic engagement is not merely nominal membership, but active and involved membership" (p. 58).

Association satisfaction remains important because of the benefits it provides to individuals. Membership in associations also appears to be related to lower levels of psychological distress (Rietschlin 1998). Tschirhart (2006) also found association membership to be tied to social and psychological benefits, such as meeting one's needs (i.e., fellowship, safety, and security) and personal awareness, growth, and improvement. Finally, Sirgy and colleagues (2000, 2001, 2010) have demonstrated that satisfaction with government and nonprofit services related positively to life and community satisfaction; however, formal associations like neighborhood or professional associations mentioned should not be the only one's included any future research.

Associations represent larger communities. Though not all associations are non-profits, many represent common classifications of non-profits (see Salomon and Anheirs 1996, Fig. 4.2). But before the invention of the not-for-profit, de Tocqueville (1966 [1988]) noted associations' abilities to draw people out of their normal groups of friends and family within communities. "Associations are historically the

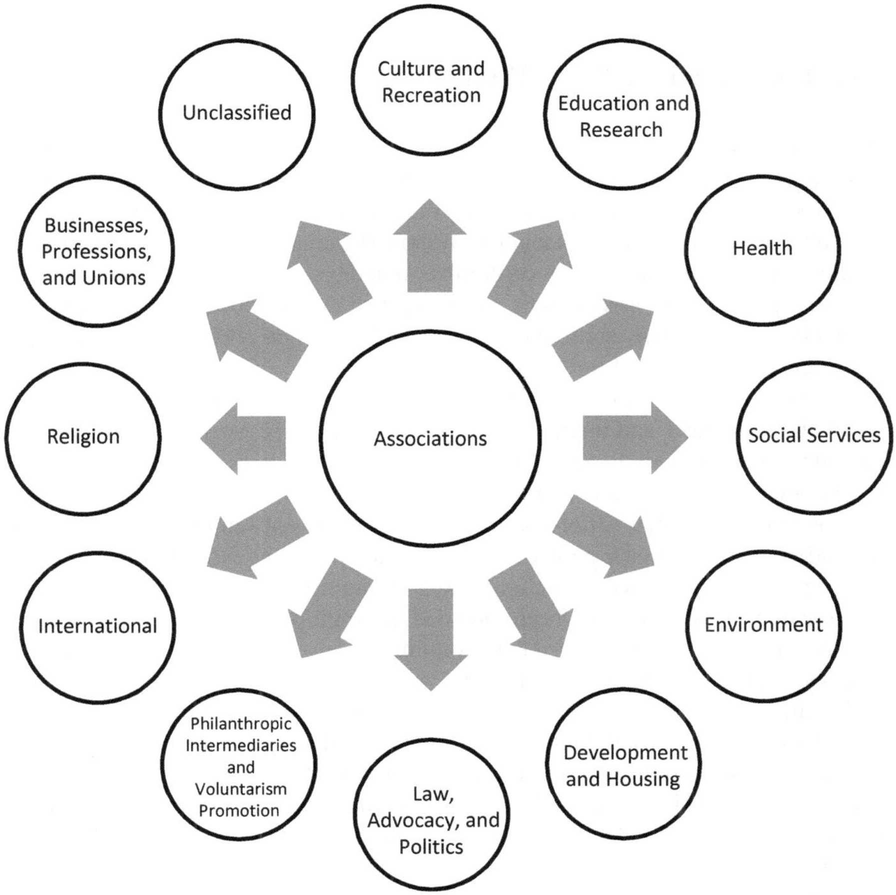

Fig. 4.2 Communities that associations represent (Adapted from Salomon and Anheir 1996)

seedbed from which the more formalized systems grow" (McKnight 2013, p. 13). Associations do not only include not-for-profit entities, though some may pursue and achieve that status (see McKnight 2013). Associations can have more horizontal and informal orientations than the typical vertically- and formally-oriented not-for-profit corporations (McKnight 2013). Incentives are likely not focused on pay (McKnight 2013); they are more intrinsic benefit-oriented as already mentioned (see Gazley and Dignam 2008, 2010). Knowledge is very much community-based as opposed to specialty-based as well (McKnight 2013). Associations are "groups of local people who came together to achieve a variety of ends... associations are groups of citizens pulled together by common consent. This consent is based upon a mutual concern or interest" (McKnight 2013, p. 2, 8). But where does this consent and interactions occur in both informal and formal associations? Thus, there is great potential for research on association events, which are often overlooked in many satisfaction models.

Event Satisfaction: What We Know So Far

If associations represent larger communities, then how are associations represented? Associations are represented by the events and persons that make them up. Events can act as societal innovations changing the relationships between the subcomponents of the association system (Rotmans 2005). Events including smaller group gatherings like committee meetings make up associations. For instance, professional associations can be broken down into individual members, committees, events (i.e. conferences), and the interactions between these components and the products of those interactions.

Researchers like Granovetter (1973, 1983) have questioned the typical line of research on linkages and interactions in social groups like associations. Too often has the research been focused on strong ties (formalized relationships), while weaker ties (informal relationships) have been overlooked. These new connections are created at and forged after associational events. Events and their successes are dependent upon the many people involved in the planning and running of events. They are the consequences of actions taken by multiple persons.

Research on events has been pursued in multiple fields such as tourism studies, tourism management studies, event management studies, and event studies (see Getz 2008); however, community and association researchers have often undervalued the role of events and event satisfaction in their fields. Citizens engage their fellow citizens and build society not just through macro-level moments (i.e. voting) but also through more micro- and meso-level small-group interaction at events (Fine and Harrington 2004). Association events have the potential to act as successful incubators of civil society through small-group interaction (Fine and Harrington 2004).

Satisfaction (and dissatisfaction) measured at association and community events has been primarily derived from consumer research (i.e. Martínez Caro and

Martinez Garcia 2007) with little intentional overlap into the community development field. Consumer research has focused on individual expectations and the setting of events (Bowen 2001; Martínez Caro and Martinez Garcia 2007). When attendees' expectations are met or exceeded, then they describe their experiences as satisfying (expectancy confirmation). When event attendees' expectations are not met, then they describe their experiences as dissatisfying (expectancy disconfirmation). Expectations focus on perceived value of items such as event program, food, location, and facility (Yoon et al. 2010).

Satisfaction (and dissatisfaction) research in organizations has started to look at organizational events. Rogelberg and colleagues (2010) found satisfaction with meetings at work related positively to job satisfaction and organizational commitment. They also found that the number of meetings that were attended moderated the relationship between meeting satisfaction and job satisfaction, such that if a person attended a large amount of meetings, then the relationship between meeting satisfaction and job satisfaction was much more salient. Finally, if meeting demands were higher, not just in quantity but in time, then the relationship was also stronger (Rogelberg et al. 2010).

Extraordinary Experiences

While events in workplaces, associations, and communities are often ordinary experiences, there is great potential for extraordinary experiences. These extremely satisfying experiences are opportunities for persons to have experiences outside of their normal ranges of choices or beyond experiences they have in their daily lives (Getz 1997; Morgan 2009). These experiences are similar to the critical incidents Herzberg and colleagues (1959) and Herzberg (1966, 1968, 1987) described.

Morgan (2009) contends that extraordinary experiences can be created and shared; thus, they can also be analyzed. Moments described as extraordinary experiences are often characterized by intense emotional or physical experiences, opportunities to increase knowledge, interactions with others, sharing of cultural values, and temporary feelings of closeness to others (Coon 1958, cited in Arnould and Price 1993; Turner 1974). Arnould and Price (1993) in their study of river rafters found extraordinary experiences to consist of thematic elements such as personal growth, self-renewal, connecting with others, and harmony with nature, all of which related to satisfaction with their experience (consistent with Whiting and Pawelko 2012).

The idea of extraordinary experiences shows natural ties to flow theory posited by Csikzentmihalyi (1997). Flow theory concerns employee absorption into work activities. Employee absorption has been shown to predict positive benefits such as employee engagement (Saks 2006). Activities that can lead to absorption or "flow" include activities with clear set goals, that provide immediate feedback, that utilize a person's skills fully, and that are moderately challenging (Csikzentmihalyi 1997). The "flow" experience can be described as losing track of time while at work and experiences of great intrinsic enjoyment (Csikzentmihalyi 1997). Looking at Walsh et al. (1985) study, the opposite of the flow experience appears troublesome when looking at feedback. Obstructing feedback from job tasks may lead to greater anxiety, lower job satisfaction, and greater intentions to leave an organization. Both "flow" experiences and feedback have been linked to Herzberg's (1966, 1987) theory (see Sachau 2007).

Herzberg and Event Satisfaction

Few studies have sought to adapt Herzberg's two-factor theory when researching event satisfaction. Researchers like Howard and Crompton (1980) have suggested that the physical attributes of tourism, parks, recreation, and special event facilities and locations parallel Herzberg's hygiene. They suggest that these attributes are necessary prerequisites for events and are already expected by event attendees much like what was discussed earlier regarding expectancy. These factors were described as necessary, but not sufficient in themselves, to create satisfying experiences for event attendees (Howard and Crompton 1980).

Howard and Crompton (1980) suggested that the motivators are primarily responsible for perceiving an event experience as positive. Motivators in leisure settings parallel the factors in the psychological environment of the event experience; however, Howard and Crompton (1980) note that the psychological environment is often highly dependent on the physical environment as well. Aspects of the psychological environment may also be positively influenced by special programing and experiences that promote an emotionally satisfying experience.

Later research by Crompton (2003) found support for the notion that events can be deconstructed into motivators and hygiene; however, in his research conducted at a large-scale city festival in the United States, these factors often overlapped. This overlap was supported by Hall et al. (2010) at a large-scale Australian festival. This overlap is also consistent with the criticism Herzberg's theory has received regarding the possible interaction between motivators and hygiene (Bockman 1971) and Herzberg's (1966) own claims that motivators do not only lead to satisfaction and hygiene does not only lead to dissatisfaction.

Crompton (2003) has suggested that there is a minimum threshold for hygiene, before motivators "emerge as satisfiers" (p. 306). The motivators described by Crompton (2003) consist of event elements that lead to social-psychological benefits. The motivators attract people to festival events and facilitate positive experiences (Crompton 2003). These factors are well-documented in Crompton and McKay's (1997) and Mohr and colleagues' (1993) reviews and displayed in Table 4.3. Many of these factors connect well with Herzberg's (1966) theory when positing these factors as antecedents to psychological growth.

Table 4.3 Reasons for attendance

Reasons	Descriptions
Cultural exploration	To experience and learn about new cultures.
Novelty and regression	To experience new things or relive old experiences.
Recover equilibrium	To help a person return to a normal affective state.
Known-group socialization	To socialize with people they already know.
External interaction or socialization	To meet and connect with new people.
Gregariousness	To do something with others.
Intellectual enrichment	To learn more in general.

Adapted from Crompton and McKay (1997) and Mohr et al. (1993)

Where Are We Now? The Search for the Community Enrichment Model

The quest for engagement in events, associations, and communities continues. As seen thus far, satisfaction has been compartmentalized into different research fields (consumer research, community development, organizational development, etc.) with the occasional overlaps. Smith (1994) noted the downfall of this compartmentalization, "Boundaries between disciplines keep us from extending our understanding" (p. 256). Additionally, involvement in associations and events has far too often been measured on one-dimensional continuums, while involvement may in fact be multidimensional (Smith 1994). Organizational theories have shown limited utility, demonstrating a "need for a new theoretical synthesis" (Knoke and Prensky 1984, p. 3). Thus, a more integrative approach is needed.

Community development researchers acknowledge communities as systems (i.e. Emery and Flora 2006; Small and Supple 2001). Small and Supple (2001) identified three components of the complex community system. The first component is the microsystems of the community consisting of families, informal groups, and associations. The second component is the relationships and linkages between individuals and these microsystems. The third component is the product of the interactions between individuals and these microsystems (Small and Supple 2001).

Associations, their events, and the individual persons involved in them have the potential to influence community capital, specifically, social capital. Increases in community capital through associations (their people and their events) may reverse the downward spiral of declining capital in communities, an aim of asset-based community development (Emery and Flora 2006). In 1957, Gunnar Myrdal posited his theory of cumulative causation, where losses in assets because of their linkages in a system will lead to further deterioration in assets. Forrester (1971) concurs with this point, "when the troubles increase, the efforts are intensified that are actually worsening the situation" (p. 115). Associations may be one integral dynamic in stopping the downward spiral.

Emery and Flora (2006) and Gutierrez-Montes (2005) found that an inverse process may exist. Emery and Flora (2006) have suggested that the best entry point into spiraling up community capital is social capital, specifically bridging capital. Associations may even be able to help communities spiral their capital up through bridging capital (Emery and Flora 2006). Associations can create new connections between heterogeneous persons and groups. These connections as mentioned earlier can be forged at community events (Fine and Harrington 2004).

The Community Enrichment Model

Therefore, a new conceptual model is proposed: A model of community enrichment (see Fig. 4.3). Enrichment is defined as personal and psychological growth modeled after Herzberg's (1966) conceptualization of psychological growth. Individuals grow from motivators such as opportunities for learning, achievement, responsibility, advancement, friendships, self-expression, fun, feedback, and recognition (Herzberg 1966; Mitchell 1983; Ewert 1994; Sachau 2007). As Sachau (2007) wrote, "The best that one can hope for is to feel contentment with or more specifically to be free from worry about hygiene" (p. 388). Hygiene includes policies, procedures, facilities, location, cost, status, security, negative social interactions, interference with one's personal life, administration, communication, and incentives (Herzberg 1966; Sachau 2007). Therefore, enrichment occurs when the minimum threshold is met, and the motivators can then come into play; this addresses criticisms regarding the interactions between hygiene and motivators (Bockman 1971; Crompton 2003).

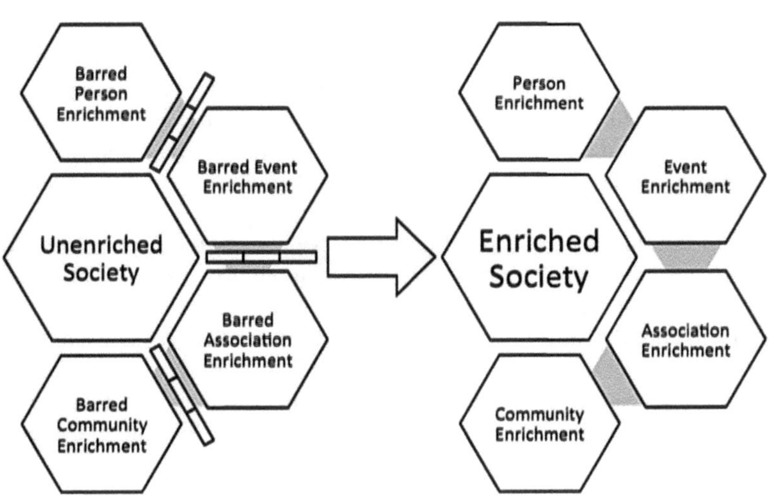

Fig. 4.3 The community enrichment model

Hygiene can be argued to parallel constraints more than motives. In Fig. 4.3, block walls represent the barring power of hygiene in an unenriched environment. Constraints are barriers that impede people from going through with their intended behaviors such as involvement in communities, associations, and events (Crawford and Godbey 1987; Crawford et al. 1991; Mannell and Kleiber 1997; Holmes and Slater 2012). Intrapersonal, interpersonal; and structural constraints, though not discussed in detail, parallel hygiene factors (Crawford and Godbey 1987; Crawford et al. 1991; Mannell and Kleiber 1997). Therefore, the removal of these barriers allows individuals to become more involved. Individuals may need to negotiate these barriers or community, association, and event leaders may need to remove them before the motivators take effect spurring greater involvement in communities, associations, and events. Thus, persons, events, associations, and communities in an enriched society work around or eliminate those barriers (see Fig. 4.3). Sure hygiene can move persons to action (see Herzberg 1966, 1968, 1987; Sachau 2007), but it is essentially more of a barrier to involvement and a driver of dissatisfaction that leads to less involvement. For instance, the location of a professional association conference may increase the likelihood of a new or current member attending the conference; however, the location may be more often indicated as the same reason the member chooses not to attend.

The motivators are where the real leverage to increase involvement exists. Motivators are posited to only have a unidirectional effect as drivers of satisfaction. Thus, the presence or increases in quality of motivators are sufficient to motivate persons to increase their involvement in the association. For example, a reason many persons attend professional association conferences is to share their work, which gives them a sense of achievement and recognition. When that work is celebrated through discussions or even awards, they are likely more driven to attend the event again or increase their involvement in the association. The absence or decreases in quality of motivators likely do not decrease involvement. A person may still want to attend a conference to present their work, even if their work is neither recognized nor celebrated. Some exceptions may occur. For example, Gazley and Dignam's (2008) study found that volunteers in professional associations were less likely to volunteer when they felt they were not thanked for their contributions. Overall, motivators do not likely act as barriers; they more likely also help in negotiating constraints.

Enrichment can occur in individuals' personal lives. Enriched persons, modeled after Herzberg's (1966) motivator seekers, are more likely to seek out events, associations, and communities that will further enrich their lives. This claim is similar to Sachau's (2007) motivational orientation, which describes individuals who are driven more by mastery-achievement and goal-achievement rather than status. The key to enrichment is the balance and value of hygiene and motivators in a person's life.

A popular adage is, "There are people who care but do not move" (Thrall 2013). These people may be motivator seekers, but hygiene constrains them from enacting their desired behaviors. The adage continues, "There are people who move but do not care" (Thrall 2013). This is a quintessential representation of hygiene seekers.

The aim of enrichment is to allow motivator seekers to be motivator seekers by removing the valuing of, dependence on, and barriers caused by hygiene, so people who care can move. A secondary aim is to alleviate the dependence on hygiene allowing people who keep moving to attain hygiene to begin to care.

Enrichment, therefore, follows a spiraling up process (see Emery and Flora 2006). Precedent for this type of spiraling process model at a micro-level can be found when looking at events, associations, and communities as systems. For example, Talmage (2013) noted that satisfaction with an event put on by the regional body of a faith-based association significantly predicted satisfaction with that regional association. Satisfaction with that event also significantly predicted satisfaction with the faith-based association as a national entity; however, that relationship was fully mediated by satisfaction with the regional body of the association.

Additional precedent can be found when viewing events as training sessions. Events can act as training sessions for association and community members instructing them on how to become better members, how to take advantage of their membership benefits (intrinsic and extrinsic, motivators and hygiene), and how to get more involved. This suggestion is consistent with Putnam's (2000) notion that associations can act as schools of democracy. Regarding satisfaction, many models of training evaluation have demonstrated its important effects (Noe 2008; Goldstein and Ford 2002).

Over 50 years ago, Donald Kirkpatrick (1959, 1960) constructed and validated one of the most widely used training evaluation models to date (Noe 2008; Goldstein and Ford 2002). Kirkpatrick's (1959, 1960, 1994) model consists of four hierarchal levels: Reactions, learning, behavior, and results. The levels overall had low intercorrelations; however, each level correlated strongly to its subsequent level (Noe 2008; Goldstein and Ford 2002). Thus, the effects of each level spiral their influence up to the next level.

Drawing on Kirkpatrick's model (1959, 1960, 1994), the enrichment model works to increase desirable behaviors and results for associations and communities. When individuals like what they experience, they learn what they can do. When they learn what they can do, they do what they want to do. When they do what they want to do, the community benefits. Thus, enrichment only occurs when the minimum threshold is hygiene met is met first, so that the motivators can take effect.

More research is needed on what defines that threshold; research on cognitive and behavioral negotiating strategies regarding constraints may be of help (see Mannell and Kleiber 1997; Jackson and Rucks 1995). Individuals that experience and value motivators may become more involved despite undesirable hygiene they may deal with. They may adjust their time management strategies to attend association and community events. The more and better quality motivators experienced, the smaller the threshold may become, but once the threshold is surpassed other benefits like learning, involvement, and overall betterment are almost sure to follow. Thus, lives can be enriched through individual extraordinary experiences, experiences at events, experiences with associations, and experiences with larger communities.

As noted thus far, satisfaction derived from motivators and dissatisfaction derived from hygiene have different effects throughout the community system, which warrants further investigation. The threshold for hygiene also needs further empirical support. But for the enrichment model to really have value, the following must be answered, "How does the diffusion of satisfaction and involvement translate into other domains as well?"

Hope lies into continued research into the internal and external reaches of social capital in community systems. Emery and Flora (2006) noted the spiraling power of social capital. Later, Geys and Murdoch (2008) noted bonding and bridging capital might be expressed both within (internally) and between (externally) associations. Likely on the individual level, the social capital of community members, association members, and event participants might hold both internal and external cognitions and behaviors (see Perkins et al. 2002) that connect them to different components of the community system. Great future insight might be gained from this notion. Thus, future research should seek answers to the questions that spring forth from the proposed enrichment model. Nonetheless, social capital still needs "to take its place in the inventory of valuable assets now dominated by measures of physical and human capital" (Schmid 2002, p. 763).

Implications for the Community

"What do people want from their communities and what components of communities are more important?" A two-factor theory provides a worthwhile approach in answering these questions. People need to have their basic needs met to avoid pain but also need to avoid boredom and experience psychological growth. If satisfaction can be seen as two-factors, then perhaps their effects may have dualities or different continuums as proposed.

Community developers and practitioners can find benefits in this way of thinking. First, policy makers can work to provide adequate services to communities in order to increase satisfaction and engagement, but realize that their efforts may only go so far. A look at presidential approval ratings in the United States helps illustrate this point. Approval ratings from Harry Truman to George W. Bush have often shown initial high ratings followed by sharp decline with a few peaks and valleys ("How the Presidents Stack Up" 2010). Thus, no matter how much change in policy is enacted by these leaders, their actions and efforts appear to have little effect on increasing satisfaction and continuous engagement. Policy makers can understand that services can only bring communities to a certain level fulfilling hygiene; thus, long-term satisfaction and engagement stems from the work of individual community members and leaders.

Community organizers are given a different charge with the two-factor approach. Aside from policy, leaders can work to facilitate or create safe environments for psychological growth. Community organizers have been very instrumental in creating community change through reaction, such as rights and suffrage movements. Thus, there is an important distinction between the efforts of organizers and policy makers. Often movements are elicited by the absence or poor quality in the fulfillment of larger community needs. The most successful movements appear to not stop at mitigating problems but also recognize and achieve sustainable and ever-adapting solutions. Successful organizers make community members feel that they individually are part of the collective that contributed to the overall success of a movement (Beckwith and Lopez 1997).

Community events, professional conferences, local celebrations, community art, and cultural experiences are worth further study and exploration. An increased knowledge of the effects of these factors may allow for significant changes in emphases for developers and leaders. For example, developers may build more or higher quality structures that may hope to facilitate continuous engagement (i.e. community art centers or cultural centers); however, they cannot stop there. To stimulate that continuous engagement, they need to find ways for community members to be involved in the decisions-made in utilizing these spaces. Additionally, neighborhood and homeowners associations may devote funds and gather community members together to create simple structures such as community signs or murals to foster community pride; however, satisfaction will be derived from the involvement of community members in the construction and design of these pieces. These associations may also hold annual gatherings or celebrations of community achievements and recognize community leaders for their efforts; thus, programs and events are created based on motivators, no longer just hygiene.

Conceptual models like the one proposed, though useful, must undergo scrutiny through empirical validation. The construction and assessment of the community enrichment model will need to use multiple methods. While the critical incidents approach has shown its worth in theory development, more testing of Herzberg's theory is needed. These questions require a mixed method approach to be properly investigated.

The best venue for further research regarding the two-factor theory is in the study of community or association events. Extraordinary experiences affect individual satisfaction and involvement in associations and communities. Many extraordinary experiences found in Herzberg's (1966, 1987) work occurred at a particular event in the workplace. Thus, community and association events can also be coded based on the presence and prevalence of Herzberg's motivators and hygiene. Qualitative studies on events may greatly benefit from using audio-video recording strategies in data collection (see Heath et al. 2010).

Questionnaires still hold merit as well. Post-event evaluations can investigate differences in satisfaction and dissatisfaction derived from motivators and hygiene. Both specific and global measures should be utilized. For instance, satisfaction may be indicated on a global measure, but dissatisfaction with a specific environmental aspect may be indicated as well (Orthner et al. 1990). Kennedy et al. (1978) have suggested that global measures are limited in their utility if not paired with specific measures. Thus, qualitative and quantitative methods and global and specific measures should be combined to test the utility of this model. Additionally, the combination of these methods helps build a strong case for trustworthiness, reliability, and validity of the new proposed model.

Conclusion

The ordinary can become extraordinary through maximizing motivators in each subcomponent of the community system and minimizing hygiene dependency and deprivation within those subcomponents. This paper has presented a new conceptual model for enriching our communities through events and associations. Heavy emphasis is placed on satisfaction. Herzberg's (1966) Two-Factor Theory is revisited in order to explore this new model and justify a resurrection of Herzberg's theory, his original theory in a new context not what it has been misunderstood to be over the past 50 years. Sachau (2007) suggests that proper resurrections of Herzberg's thinking should not be in refabricating or retesting his theory but should be used when understanding his work, "as a general framework for understanding the dual nature of satisfaction/dissatisfaction" (p. 389). Today, Herzberg's work still appears meritorious as a meta-theoretical approach or framework than the prescriptive theory that was once used. His Two-Factor Theory aims to better the lives of individuals (a goal we all hopefully share), so that their individual environments may also be bettered or, as Herzberg (1987) termed, enriched.

Acknowledgements Craig Talmage wishes to recognize the on-going support of his mentor Dr. Richard Knopf who has challenged him to seek excellence in teaching and research. He wishes to thank Mikulas Pstross for his listening ear and careful eye through many versions of this work. He also thanks Daniel Sachau for his strive to keep Herzberg's framework alive in his teaching and research. He is grateful for all his family and friends that continue to support him as he seeks to find the elements of our communities and relationships that drive us to be better.

References

Adler, R. P., & Goggin, J. (2005). What do we mean by "civic engagement"? *Journal of Transformative Education, 3*(3), 236–253.

Albert, L. R., & Dignam, M. (2010). *The decision to learn: Why people seek continuing education and how membership organizations can meet learners needs.* Washington, DC: ASAE: The Center for Association Leadership.

Allen, L. R., Long, P. T., & Perdue, R. R. (1991). Relational patterns between community dimensions and global measures of community satisfaction. *Journal of Rural Studies, 7*(3), 331–338.

Amérigo, M., & Aragonés, J. I. (1988). Satisfaccion residencial en un barrio remodeládo: Predictores fisicos y sociales. *Revista de Psicologia Social, 3*, 61–70.

Amérigo, M., & Aragonés, J. I. (1990). Residential satisfaction in council housing. *Journal of Environmental Psychology, 10*, 313–325.

Arnould, E. J., & Price, L. L. (1993). River magic: Extraordinary experience and the extended service encounter. *Journal of Consumer Research, 20*, 24–35.

Bach, R. L. & Smith, J. (1977, May). Community satisfaction, expectations of moving, and migration. *Demography, 14*(2), 147–167.
Bassett-Jones, N., & Lloyd, G. C. (2005). Does Herzberg's motivation theory have staying power? *The Journal of Management Development, 24*(10), 929–943.
Beckwith, D., & Lopez, C. (1997). *Community organizing: People power from the grassroots*. Washington, DC: Center for Community Change.
Belias, D., & Koustelios, A. (2014). Organizational culture and job satisfaction: A review. *International Review of Management and Marketing, 4*(2), 132–149.
Bellah, R. N., Madsen, R., Sullivan, W., Swidler, A., & Tipton, S. (1985). *Habits of the heart: Individualism and commitment in American life*. Berkeley: University of California Press.
Bleuel, B. (1990). Customer dissatisfaction and the zone of uncertainty. *Journal of Services Marketing, 4*(1), 49–52.
Block, M., & Zautra, A. (1981). Satisfaction and distress in community: A test of the effects of life events. *American Journal of Community Psychology, 9*(2), 165–180.
Bockman, V. M. (1971). The Herzberg controversy. *Personnel Psychology, 24*, 155–189.
Bowen, D. (2001). Antecedents of consumer satisfaction and dis-satisfaction (CS/D) on long-haul inclusive tours—A reality check on theoretical considerations. *Tourism Management, 22*(1), 49–61.
Brackertz, N., & Kenley. (2002). Evaluating community facilities in local government: Managing for service enablement. *Journal of Facilities Management, 1*(3), 283–299.
Brown, R. B. (1993). Rural community satisfaction and attachment in mass consumer society. *Rural Sociology, 58*, 387–403.
Buttel, F. H., Martinson, O. B., & Wilkening, E. A. (1979). Size of place and community attachment: A reconsideration. *Social Indicators Research, 6*(4), 475–485.
Caldwell, L. L., & Andereck, K. L. (1994). Motives for initiating and continuing membership in a recreation-related voluntary association. *Leisure Sciences, 16*, 33–44.
Campbell, A., Converse, P. E., & Rodgers, W. L. (1976). *The quality of American life*. New York: Russell Sage.
Carvalho, C., Brito, C., & Cabral, J. S. (2010). Towards a conceptual model for assessing the quality of public services. *International Review on Public and Nonprofit Marketing, 7*(1), 69–86.
Coon, C. (1958). *Caravan: The story of the middle east*. New York: Holt, Rinehart.
Costa, D. L., & Kahn, M. E. (2004). Civic engagement and community heterogeneity: An economist's perspective. *Perspectives on Politics, 1*(01), 103–111.
Crawford, D. W., & Godbey, G. (1987). Reconceptualizing barriers to family leisure. *Leisure Sciences, 9*(2), 119–127.
Crawford, D. W., Jackson, E. L., & Godbey, G. (1991). A hierarchical model of leisure constraints. *Leisure Sciences, 13*(4), 309–320.
Crompton, J. L. (2003). Adapting Herzberg: A conceptualization of the effects of hygiene and motivator attributes on perceptions of event quality. *Journal of Travel Research, 41*(3), 305–310.
Crompton, J. L., & McKay, S. L. (1997). Motives of visitors attending festival events. *Annals of Tourism Research, 24*(2), 425–439.
Csikzentmihalyi, M. (1997). *Finding flow: The psychology of engagement in everyday life*. New York: Basic Books.
Dalton, J., & Dignam, M. (2007). *The decision to join: How individuals determine value and why they choose to belong*. Washington, DC: ASAE & The Center for Association Leadership.
Dawes, J., & Rowley, J. (1999). Negative evaluations of service quality-a framework for identification and response. *Journal of Marketing Practice: Applied Marketing Science, 5*(2), 46–55.
de Tocqueville, A. [1988 (1966)]. *Democracy in America*. New York: Harper & Row.
Deci, E. L., & Ryan, R. M. (1985). *Intrinsic motivation and self-determination in human behavior*. New York: Plenum.
Emery, M., & Flora, C. (2006). Spiraling-up: Mapping community transformation with community capitals framework. *Community Development, 37*(1), 19–35.

Ewert, A. W. (1994). Playing the edge: Motivation and risk taking in a high-altitude wilderness-like environment. *Environment and Behavior, 26*, 3–24.

Filkins, R., Allen, J. C., & Cordes, S. (2000). Predicting community satisfaction among rural residents: An integrative model. *Rural Sociology, 65*(1), 72–86.

Findlay, J. N. (1967). *Values and intentions: A study in value theory and philosophy*. New York: Humanities Press.

Fine, G. A., & Harrington, B. (2004). Tiny publics: Small groups and civil society. *Sociological Theory, 22*(3), 341–356.

Forrester, J. W. (1971). Counterintuitive behavior of social systems. *Theory and Decision, 2*(2), 109–140.

Fried, M. (1982). Residential attachment: Sources of residential and community satisfaction. *Journal of Social Issues, 38*(3), 107–119.

Fuguitt, G. V., & Zuiches, J. J. (1975). Residential preferences and population distribution. *Demography, 12*(3), 491–504.

Gazley, B. A., & Dignam, M. (2008). *The decision to volunteer*. Washington, DC: ASAE and The Center for Association Leadership.

Gazley, B. A., & Dignam, M. (2010). *The decision to give*. Washington, DC: ASAE and The Center for Association Leadership.

Getz, D. (1997). *Event management & event tourism*. New York: Cognizant Communication Corp.

Getz, D. (2008). Event tourism: Definition, evolution, and research. *Tourism Management, 29*(3), 403–428.

Geys, B., & Murdoch, Z. (2008). How to make head or tail of 'bridging' and 'bonding'?: Addressing the methodological ambiguity. *The British Journal of Sociology, 59*(3), 435–454.

Goldstein, I. L., & Ford, J. K. (2002). *Training in organizations: Needs assessment, development, and evaluation* (4th ed.). Belmont: Wadsworth Group.

Goudy, W. J. (1977). Evaluations of local attributes and community satisfaction in small towns. *Rural Sociology, 42*, 371–382.

Granovetter, M. S. (1973). The strength of weak ties. *American Journal of Sociology, 78*(6), 1360–1380.

Granovetter, M. S. (1983). The strength of weak ties: A network theory revisited. *Sociological Theory, 1*(1), 201–233.

Grillo, M. C., Teixeira, M. A., & Wilson, D. C. (2010). Residential satisfaction and civic engagement: Understanding the causes of community participation. *Social Indicators Research, 97*, 451–466.

Gutierrez-Montes, I. (2005). *Healthy communities equals healthy ecosystems? Evolution (and breakdown) of a participatory ecological research project towards a community natural resource management process, San Miguel Chimalapa (Mexico).* PhD dissertation, Iowa State University, Ames.

Hall, J., Basarin, V. J., & Lockstone-Binney, L. (2010). An empirical analysis of attendance at a commemorative event: Anzac Day at Gallipoli. *International Journal of Hospitality Management, 29*(2), 245–253.

Heath, C., Hindmarsh, J., & Luff, P. (2010). *Video in qualitative research: Analysing social interactions in everyday life*. London: Sage Publications Ltd.

Heaton, T., Fredrickson, C., Fuguitt, G. V., & Zuiches, J. J. (1979). Residential preferences, community satisfaction, and the intention to move. *Demography, 16*(4), 565–573.

Herzberg, F. (1966). *Work and nature of man*. New York: Mentor Books.

Herzberg, F. I. (1968). One more time: How do you motivate employees? *Harvard Business Review, 46*(1), 53–62.

Herzberg, F. (1974). Motivation-hygiene profiles. *Organizational Dynamics, 3*(2), 18–29.

Herzberg, F. I. (1987). One more time: How do you motivate employees? *Harvard Business Review, 65*(5), 109–120, including a retrospective commentary. (Reprint from 1968)

Herzberg, F. I., Mausner, R., Peterson, R., & Capwell, D. (1957). *Job attitudes: Review of research and opinion*. Pittsburgh: Psychological Services of Pittsburgh.

Herzberg, F. I., Mausner, B., & Snyderman, B. (1959). *The motivation to work* (2nd ed.). New York: Wiley.

Holmes, K., & Slater, A. (2012). Patterns of voluntary participation in membership associations: A study of UK heritage supporter groups. *Nonprofit and Voluntary Sector Quarterly, 41*(5), 850–869.

"How the Presidents Stack Up". (2010). *Wall Street Journal Online.* Available Online 15 November, 2010 at: http://online.wsj.com/public/resources/documents/info-presapp0605-31.html

Howard, D. R., & Crompton, J. L. (1980). *Financing, managing and marketing recreation and park resources.* Dubuque: William C. Brown.

Hughey, J. B., & Bardo, J. W. (1984). The structure of community satisfaction in a Southeastern American city. *Journal of Social Psychology, 123*(1), 91–99.

Ikeda, K. I., Kobayashi, T., & Hoshimoto, M. (2008). Does political participation make a difference? The relationship between political choice, civic engagement and political efficacy. *Electoral Studies, 27*(1), 77–88.

Iso-Ahola, S. E. (1980). *The social psychology of leisure and recreation.* Dubuque: Wm. C. Brown Company Publishers.

Jackson, E. L., & Rucks, V. C. (1995). Negotiation of leisure constraints by junior-high and high-school students: An exploratory study. *Journal of Leisure Research, 27*, 85–105.

Johnson 2013, P. (2013, May 7). Panel discussion. *Together: Building the Arizona we want.* Phoenix: Experience Matters.

Johnston, R. (1995). The zone of tolerance: Exploring the relationship between service transactions and satisfaction with the overall service. *International Journal of Service Industry Management, 6*(2), 46–61.

Kaplan, R. (1984). Impact of urban nature: A theoretical analysis. *Urban Ecology, 8*, 189–197.

Kaplan, R. (2001). The nature of the view from home: Psychological benefits. *Environmental Behavior, 33*, 507–542.

Kennedy, L. W., Northcott, H. C., & Kiazel, C. (1978). Subjective evaluation of well-being: Problems and prospects. *Social Indicators Research, 5*, 451–474.

King, D. C., & Walker, J. L. (1992). The provision of benefits by interest groups in the United States. *Journal of Politics, 54*, 394–426.

Kirkpatrick, D. L. (1959, 1960). Techniques for evaluating training programs. *Journal of the American Society of Training Directors, 13*, 3–32.

Kirkpatrick, D. L. (1994). *Evaluating training programs: The four levels.* San Francisco: Berrett-Koehler.

Knack, S., & Keefer, P. (2003). *Does social capital have an economic payoff? Democracy, governance, and growth.* Ann Arbor: University of Michigan Press.

Knoke, D., & Prensky, D. (1984). What relevance do organization theories have for voluntary associations? *Social Science Quarterly, 65*(1), 3–20.

Lewin, K. L. (1931). Environmental forces in child behavior and development. In C. Murchison (Ed.), *A handbook of child psychology.* Worcester: Clark University Press.

Mannell, R. C., & Kleiber, D. A. (1997). *A social psychology of leisure.* State College: Venture Publishing, Inc.

Martinez Caro, L., & Martinez Garcia, J. A. (2007). Cognitive–affective model of consumer satisfaction. An exploratory study within the framework of a sporting event. *Journal of Business Research, 60*(2), 108–114.

Maslow, A. H. (1954). *Motivation and personality.* New York: Harper.

McKnight, J. (1987). Regenerating community. *Social Policy, 17*(3), 54–58.

McKnight, J. (2013). *The four-legged stool.* Dayton: The Kettering Foundation.

Medalia, N. Z. (1964). Air pollution as a socio-environmental health problems: A survey report. *Journal of Health and Human Behavior, 5*(4), 154–165.

Miller, F. D., Tsemberis, S., Malia, G. P., & Grega, D. (1980). Neighborhood satisfaction among urban dwellers. *Journal of Social Issues, 36*(3), 101–117.

Mitchell, R. G. (1983). *Mountain experience: The psychology and sociology of adventure.* Chicago: The University of Chicago Press.

Mohr, K., Backman, K. F., Gahan, L. W., & Backman, S. J. (1993). An investigation of festival motivations and event satisfaction by visitor type. *Festival Management and Event Tourism, 1*, 89–97.

Molnar, J. J., Purohit, S., Clonts, H. A., & Lee, V. W. (1979). A longitudinal analysis of satisfaction with selected community services in a nonmetropolitan area. *Rural Sociology, 44*(2), 401–419.

Morgan, M. (2009). What makes a good festival? Understanding the event experience. *Event Management, 12*(2), 81–93.

Myrdal, G. (1957). *Economic theory and underdeveloped regions*. London: Duckworth.

Noe, R. A. (2008). *Employee training and development* (4th ed.). New York: McGraw-Hill Irwin.

Oliver, R. L. (1997). *Satisfaction: A behavioral perspective on the consumer*. New York: McGraw Hill.

Orthner, D. K., Esther, D., & Stawarski, C. (1990). *Community satisfaction: Implications for army communities. ARI Research Note 90–96*. United States Army Research Institute for the Behavioral and Social Sciences. Chapel Hill: North Carolina

Payne, L. L., & Schaumleffel, N. A. (2008). Relationship between attitudes toward rural community parks and recreation and rural community satisfaction. *Journal of Park and Recreation Administration, 26*(3), 116–135.

Pennell, F. E. (1978). Collective vs. private strategies for coping with crime: The consequences for citizen perceptions of crime, attitudes toward the police and neighboring activity. *Nonprofit and Voluntary Sector Quarterly, 7*(1–2), 59–74.

Perkins, D. D., Hughey, J., & Speer, P. W. (2002). Community psychology perspectives on social capital theory and community development practice. *Community Development, 33*(1), 33–52.

Putnam, R. D. (1995). Bowling alone: America's declining social capital. *Journal of Democracy, 6*, 65–78.

Putnam, R. D. (2000). *Bowling alone: The collapse and revival of American community*. New York: Simon & Schuster.

Rietschlin, J. (1998). Voluntary association membership and psychological distress. *Journal of Health and Social Behavior, 39*, 349–355.

Rodgers, W. (1980). Residential satisfaction in relationships to size of place. *Social Psychology Quarterly, 13*(4), 236–441.

Rogelberg, S. G., Allen, J. A., Shanock, L., Scott, C., & Shuffler, M. (2010). Employee satisfaction with meetings: A contemporary facet of job satisfaction. *Human Resource Management, 49*(2), 149–172.

Rossi, P. H. (1955). *Why families move: A study in the social psychology of urban residential mobility*. New York: The Free Press.

Rotmans, J. (2005). *Societal innovation: Between dream and reality lies complexity* (Inaugural addresses research in management series). Rotterdam: Erasmus University Rotterdam.

Sachau, D. A. (2007). Resurrecting the motivation-hygiene theory: Herzberg and the positive psychology movement. *Human Resource Development Review, 6*(4), 377–393.

Saks, A. M. (2006). Antecedents and consequences of employee engagement. *Journal of Managerial Psychology, 21*(7), 600–619.

Salamon, L. M., & Anheier, H. K. (1996). *The International Classification of Nonprofit Organizations: ICNPO-Revision 1, 1996* (The Johns Hopkins Comparative Nonprofit Sector Project: Working Paper No. 19). Baltimore: The Johns Hopkins Institute for Policy Studies.

Sampson, R. J. (1991). Linking the micro- and macro-level dimensions of community social organization. *Social Forces, 70*(1), 43–64.

Schmid, A. A. (2002). Using motive to distinguish social capital from its outputs. *Journal of Economic Issues, 36*(3), 747–768.

Schulze, R., Artis, J., & Beegle, J. A. (1963). The measurement of community satisfaction and the decision to migrate. *Rural Sociology, 28*, 279–283.

Scitovsky, I. (1976). *The joyless economy: An inquiry into human satisfaction and dissatisfaction*. New York: Oxford University Press.

Sirgy, M. J., & Cornwell, T. (2001). Further validation of Sirgy et al.'s measure of community quality of life. *Social Indicators Research, 56*, 125–143.
Sirgy, M. J., Rahtz, D. R., Cicic, M., & Underwood, R. (2000). A method for assessing residents' satisfaction with community-based services: A quality-of-life perspective. *Social Indicators Research, 49*, 279–316.
Sirgy, M. J., Widgery, R. N., Lee, D., & Yu, G. B. (2010). Developing a measure of community well-being based on perceptions of impact in various life domains. *Social Indicators Research, 96*, 295–311.
Slater, A. (2003). Users or supporters? Understanding the motivations and behaviors of members. *Curator: The Museum Journal, 46*, 182–207.
Small, S., & Supple, A. (2001). Communities as systems: Is a community more than the sum of its parts. In A. Booth & A. C. Crouter (Eds.), *Does it take a village? Community effects on children, adolescents, and families* (pp. 159–187). Mahwah: Lawrence Erlbaum Associates, Inc.
Smith, D. H. (1994). Determinants of voluntary association participation and volunteering: A literature review. *Nonprofit and Voluntary Sector Quarterly, 23*(3), 243–263.
Smith, E. R., & Miller, F. D. (1978). Limits on perception of cognitive processes: A reply to Nisbett and Wilson. *Psychological Review, 85*, 355–362.
Speare, A., Jr. (1974). Residential satisfaction as an intervening variable in residential mobility. *Demography, 11*(2), 173–188.
Sutaria, R. (1980). Personality, needs and two-factor theory of work motivation. *Indian Journal of Industrial Relations, 16*(2), 219–223.
Talmage, C. (2013). Community enrichment report: A study of the 2013 synod assembly. *Arizona State University's Partnership for Community Development*. Technical report. Phoenix: Arizona
Thrall, B. (2013, June 4). *Weekly partnership for community development meeting*. Phoenix: Arizona State University.
Tschirhart, M. (2006). Nonprofit membership associations. In W. W. Powell & R. Steinberg (Eds.), *The nonprofit sector: A research handbook* (pp. 523–541). New Haven: Yale University Press.
Turner, V. W. (1974). Social drama and ritual metaphors. In *Dramas, fields and metaphors* (pp. 23–59). Ithaca: Cornell University Press.
Vreugdenhil, A., & Rigby, K. (1987). Assessing generalized community satisfaction. *The Journal of Social Psychology, 127*(4), 367–374.
Wagner, R., & Harter, J. K. (2006). *12 elements of great managing*. New York: Gallup Press.
Walsh, J. P., Ashford, S. J., & Hill, T. E. (1985). Feedback obstruction: The influence of the information environment on employee turnover intentions. *Human Relations, 38*(1), 23–46.
White, P. (1980). Limitations on verbal reports of internal events: A refutation of Nisbett and Wilson and of Bem. *Psychological Review, 87*, 105–112.
White, M. J. (1985). Determinants of community satisfaction in Middletown. *American Journal of Community Psychology, 13*(5), 583–597.
Whiting, J. W., & Pawelko, K. A. (2012). *A naturalistic inquiry into the social world of whitewater kayakers. Notes*. In Proceedings of the 2010 Northeastern recreation research symposium. U.S. Forest Service Northern Research Station Newtown Square, PA.
Wollebaek, D., & Selle, P. (2002). Does participation in voluntary associations contribute to social capital? The impact of intensity, scope, and type. *Nonprofit and Voluntary Sector Quarterly, 31*(1), 32–61.
Wollebaek, D., & Selle, P. (2003). The importance of passive membership. In M. Hooghe & D. Stolle (Eds.), *Generating social capital: Civil society and institutions in comparative perspective* (pp. 67–88). New York: Palgrave Macmillan.
Yoon, Y. S., Lee, J. S., & Lee, C. K. (2010). Measuring festival quality and value affecting visitors' satisfaction and loyalty using a structural approach. *International Journal of Hospitality Management, 29*(2), 335–342.
Zehner, R. B. (1971). Neighborhood and community satisfaction in new towns and less planned suburbs. *Journal of the American Planning Association, 37*(6), 379–385.

Chapter 5
Explaining the Ethnic Minority Disadvantage in Subjective Well-Being: A Multilevel Analysis of European Countries

Thomas de Vroome and Marc Hooghe

Introduction

Social inequality is one of the classic problems studied in sociology (Lenski 1966). The research on social inequality and stratification has broadened from a focus on class divisions in society to a focus including the dividing lines of race and ethnicity, which often intersect with class divisions (Anthias 2001). Consequently, many studies have provided evidence for the disadvantaged position of ethnic minorities in societies, mainly focusing on economic indicators such as employment and income (De Jong and Madamba 2001; Rooth and Ekberg 2003; Van Tubergen 2006).

More recently, psychologists have argued that measures of subjective well-being, such as life satisfaction and happiness, can be important additional indicators of inequality in society (Diener 2000; Veenhoven 2004). Measures of subjective well-being can be an important addition to traditional economic indicators of inequality, because they more closely reflect what people themselves find important in life (Veenhoven 2004). When research can show evidence for determinants of subjective well-being, then policies could be developed that improve quality of life from the perspectives of citizens themselves.

Research has shown that subjective well-being encompasses distinct components, with the clearest distinction being made between life satisfaction, on the one hand, and happiness on the other (Angner 2010). Life satisfaction is the more cognitive component of subjective well-being, and can be defined as people's evaluations and judgments about their quality of life as a whole, while happiness is the more experiential component, which can be defined as people's feelings about whether they are generally in a positive mood (Angner 2010; Diener 2000). In this

T. de Vroome (✉) • M. Hooghe
ERCOMER, Utrecht University, Postbus 80.140, 3508 TC Utrecht, Netherlands
e-mail: T.M.deVroome@uu.nl; Marc.Hooghe@soc.kuleuven.be

F. Maggino (ed.), *A New Research Agenda for Improvements in Quality of Life*, Social Indicators Research Series 57, DOI 10.1007/978-3-319-15904-1_5

study, we focus on both of these important aspects of subjective well-being. We investigate the differences in subjective well-being between ethnic minorities and majority members in European societies.

Previous research on immigrant populations strongly suggests that levels of subjective well-being are lower among ethnic minorities than among majority group members. A cross-national study among first and second generation immigrants in 13 European countries showed that life satisfaction and happiness were lower among these groups, compared to natives (Safi 2010). Several national studies on immigrant populations showed similar results, across different destination countries in Western Europe and different immigrant origin countries, such as from Eastern Europe, Asian and African countries (Bălţătescu 2007; De Vroome and Hooghe 2013; Verkuyten 2008).

Importantly, however, these previous studies in Europe have focused on minorities with an immigrant background, rather than on ethnic minorities. The distinction is crucial, because ethnic minorities can also include indigenous minorities. Moreover, the terms 'immigrant' and 'second generation immigrant' are becoming increasingly contested when it comes to the descendants of immigrants, because the terms itself can have a stigmatizing effect, on the one hand, and because individuals whose families have settled in a country more than two generations ago can still consider themselves as members of an ethnic minority group, on the other (Ahmed et al. 2007; Thomassen 2010). In this study, therefore, we focus on self-defined ethnic minority status, whether this status is related to immigration history or experience or not.

The aim of this study is to explain the gap in subjective well-being between those citizens who define themselves as a member of an ethnic minority group and those who define themselves as a member of the majority population. To explain this gap, we use the need-gratification theory, which is based on Maslow's theory of human motivation (Oishi et al. 1999). From this perspective, we make the connection between the economically disadvantaged position and experiences of discrimination among minority group members, on the one hand, and their lower levels of life satisfaction and happiness, on the other. We investigate both whether economic position and perceived discrimination can explain the gap in subjective well-being between majority and minority members, and to what extent economic position and discrimination have a similar effect on subjective well-being among these groups.

To answer our research questions, we use the fifth edition of the European Social Survey (ESS), which was administered over the course of 2010 and 2011. These data allow us to conduct a multilevel analysis of subjective well-being among majority and minority members across 20 European countries.

Economic Position, Discrimination and Need-Gratification

Need-gratification theory is especially well-equipped to study the differences in subjective well-being that can be observed between members of the native majority and those who define themselves as ethnic minorities. The need-gratification approach argues that subjective well-being is based on the extent to which universal human needs are fulfilled. These needs include basic physiological needs such as food and water, the needs for a sense of safety, love and belonging, esteem and positive regard, and the desire for personal growth (Maslow 1970; Oishi et al. 1999; Veenhoven 1991).

Many studies have shown that, on average, minority groups in Western societies are facing disadvantaged socio-economic positions (Nazroo 2003; Van Tubergen 2006). Moreover, these socio-economic disadvantages have been convincingly shown to be associated with inequalities in health, which can also be considered an important component of quality of life (Cooper 2002; Nazroo 2003). These medical studies further suggest that socio-economic disadvantage can frustrate the gratification of physiological needs. Moreover, economic position can be related to the needs for esteem and personal growth, as professional activities are a clear source of respect and an outlet for creativity. The perception of discrimination, on the other hand, can be negatively related to the need for esteem and a sense of belonging, and can furthermore threaten individuals' sense of safety. Because members of ethnic minority groups have often been found to hold disadvantaged socio-economic positions in Western societies, and because minority group members are likely to perceive higher levels of discrimination than majority members, we focus on these two factors to explain majority-minority differences in subjective well-being.

Economic Position

Economic position is one of the most important explanations of subjective well-being that has been investigated in previous research. Especially among those who occupy the lower positions on the socio-economic ladder, research has shown that access to material resources can have a strong impact on subjective well-being (Cheung and Leung 2004). For those who occupy the lower socio-economic strata, increments in economic position can mean that more of the basic human needs can be fulfilled, and a sense of safety can be improved by, for instance, higher quality housing and reduced employment insecurity. Among those who find themselves in the higher socio-economic strata of society, the effect of an increase in economic resources is much more modest, as this will have much less of a marginal effect on their opportunities to satisfy basic human needs (Cheung and Leung 2004).

Relatedly, the extent to which income has a positive effect on subjective well-being is fiercely debated in the literature. Studies on the relation between income and subjective well-being often find a positive but rather weak effect (Headey et al. 2004; Moghaddam 2008). This is due to the fact that, as one moves higher up on the income distribution, the effects on subjective well-being become increasingly small or non-existent. From the perspective of need-gratification theory, therefore, it is necessary to assess the impact of economic position with additional measures that are qualitatively different from the income operationalization. Unemployment and economic inactivity can deny people the opportunity for a professional source of positive regard, interpersonal contact, and self-actualization, while participation in higher education can have the reverse effect. Moreover, measures that more directly tap people's experience of economic well-being may show a much clearer relation between economic position and subjective well-being than a measure of income (Moghaddam 2008). Especially among minority group members, measures of job satisfaction and experienced financial problems can be very relevant, as underemployment and financial insecurity are likely much more prevalent among these groups (De Jong and Madamba 2001; Slack and Jensen 2002). The expectations on economic disadvantage among ethnic minority members and the relation between economic position and subjective well-being lead to the following hypothesis:

H1. The differences in subjective well-being between majority group members and ethnic minorities can be explained by differences in economic position.

Perceived Discrimination

Zick et al. (2008) have noted that ethnic discrimination does remain a widespread problem throughout Europe. Partly as a reaction, minority individuals show lower national attachment, or in other words a more negative attitude towards society (Jasinskaja-Lahti et al. 2009). This means that discrimination is associated with reduced feelings of belonging, which can in turn have a negative impact on subjective well-being.

In relation, there is already research evidence available demonstrating the relation between perceived discrimination among minority groups and subjective well-being. Safi (2010) has concluded on the basis of a cross-national study in European countries that discrimination is perhaps the most consistent correlate of life satisfaction among first and second generation immigrants. Other studies, in Europe and Canada, have also indicated a strong relation between perceived discrimination and subjective well-being among immigrant groups (Verkuyten 2008; Vohra and Adair 2000).

Regarding ethnic minority groups, research in a US context shows similar results. Studies among African American, Asian American and Latino American individuals indicate that discrimination significantly reduces quality of life outcomes among ethnic minority groups (Branscombe et al. 1999; Utsey et al. 2002). Beyond the frustration of a need for belonging, the mechanisms in the relation between perceived discrimination and subjective well-being include decreased personal and group self-esteem, and heightened stress and decreased mental health (Cassidy et al. 2004; Williams et al. 2003). Though discrimination does not only occur on ethno-racial, cultural or religious grounds, but can also focus on characteristics such as gender, age, sexual preference or disability, it can be expected that members of ethnic minority groups perceive more discrimination in society than members of majority groups. Therefore, our second hypothesis is the following:

H2. The differences in subjective well-being between majority group members and ethnic minorities can be explained by differences in experienced discrimination.

Do Economic Position and Discrimination Equally Affect Majority Members?

Our main argument is that economic position and perceived discrimination can have a mediating role, meaning that they can possibly explain differences between minority and majority group members in subjective well-being. However, we also want to explore the extent to which economic position and discrimination have a different impact on subjective well-being among majority group members than they have among members of minority populations, in other words the interaction effects.

Because the effects of discrimination, and to a lesser extent economic position, have often been studied from within a discourse of minority disadvantage, one could ask whether these factors are equally important for the subjective well-being of those who consider themselves a member of the majority in their country. Moreover, previous research suggests that the explanations of subjective well-being can differ between countries and cross-culturally, and between social groups defined by class positions (Cheung and Leung 2004; Diener and Diener 1995; Oishi et al. 1999).

Regarding the effects of income, recent studies suggests that minority groups may benefit more from income mobility, in terms of their subjective well-being, than members of majority populations (Bartram 2011; Olgiati et al. 2013). This can be related to the economically disadvantaged position of minority communities in most societies. Need-gratification theory suggests that gratification of the more basic needs, such as nutrition and safety, takes precedence over gratification of the higher order needs such as esteem and self-actualization (Oishi et al. 1999). For minority group members, incremental improvements in economic position may be more strongly related to the lower-order physiological and safety needs of both themselves, but also of their wider social circle, thereby having a relatively greater impact on subjective well-being.

A similar argument can be made regarding the effect of perceived discrimination on subjective well-being. In principle, being discriminated against can be expected to have a negative impact on subjective well-being for all members of society, and our main argument implies simply that minority group members will encounter more discrimination than majority group members. However, a sense of collective identity may be especially salient and directly related to subjective well-being among ethnic minority groups, relative to other discriminated groups in society such as women, elderly people or the disabled. Indeed, research shows a strong relation between discrimination and collective self-esteem among minority groups, suggesting that social identity mechanisms may be especially relevant for ethnic minority individuals compared to other discriminated individuals in society (Cassidy et al. 2004). Our third hypothesis is therefore that:

H3. The effects of economic position and experienced discrimination on subjective well-being will be stronger among ethnic minorities than among majority group members.

Data and Methods

Our analysis is based on the fifth edition of the European Social Survey, with supplemental country level data, which is necessary for our multilevel approach. The data applied here is based on the ESS Multilevel Data Repository. The individual level data is taken from the surveys that have been administered over the course of 2010 and 2011, in 27 European countries in total. The country level data is provided by Eurostat and the OECD, and prepared and made publicly available by the Norwegian Social Science Data Services (NSD).

Because country level living conditions are important to take into account from the perspective of need gratification theory, only the 20 countries for which the additional macro data was available from Eurostat and the OECD were included in the analysis presented here. These countries are Belgium, Switzerland, the Czech Republic, Germany, Denmark, Estonia, Spain, Finland, France, United Kingdom, Greece, Hungary, Ireland, the Netherlands, Norway, Poland, Portugal, Sweden, Slovenia and Slovakia. We have deleted cases with missing values listwise, with two exceptions discussed below. All in all, our analyses are therefore based on a sample that includes 36,969 respondents.

The ESS data have some great advantages for the purpose of the present paper, as they include a broad selection of European countries, measures of two important components of subjective well-being, and sufficient information on individual and household economic positions. However, due to time and budget limitations, a disadvantage is that most constructs were measured with only a limited number of items, frequently only one survey question. Moreover, due to the fact that minority groups were not intentionally oversampled, as is done in many national and experimental studies on migration issues, the number of respondents that self-identify as member of a minority group is relatively low. Our sample contains 1,586 minority group members, which does not allow extensive country level comparisons. Therefore, we take the most important country level control variables into account, but focus on individual level theoretical explanations.

It is also worthwhile to note that the number of respondents who self-identify as a member of an ethnic minority group is about half the number of the respondents that are foreign-born, and about a quarter of the respondents that are either foreign born or would be classified as second generation immigrants (people of whom one or both parents are foreign-born). This underlines the fact that part of the foreign-born and 'second-generation immigrants' originate from families that once already lived in the current country of residence, in other words have returned to the country of their ancestors, and that these and other people who would externally be classified as a first or second generation immigrant do not necessarily consider themselves a member of an ethnic minority group. In fact, slightly more than a third of first generation immigrants and only slightly more than a tenth of the second generation immigrants in our sample self-identify as ethnic minority group member. Conversely about a third of the respondents in our sample who self-identify as an ethnic minority group member would externally be classified as natives, which means that this group is made up of indigenous minorities or descendants of migrants from more than two generations ago (see Appendix Table A.1).

Dependent Variables

The ESS survey has two questions on subjective well-being, one addressing life satisfaction and the other addressing happiness. The variable for life satisfaction was measured with the question: 'All things considered, how satisfied are you with your life as a whole nowadays?'. The variable for happiness was measured with the question: 'Taking all things together, how happy would you say you are?'. Both questions were answered on 11-point scales, running from 0 (extremely dissatisfied/unhappy) to 10 (extremely satisfied/happy).

Independent Variables

The crucial independent variable for our analysis is self-identification as member of an ethnic minority group. This variable was measured with the question: 'Do you belong to a minority ethnic group in [country]?'. Respondents could answer to this question by replying 'yes' or 'no'.

We use three objective indicators of economic position. First, we use a measure of current employment status, with four categories, distinguishing those respondents who are currently in paid employment, from students, people who are unemployed and looking for work, and people who are inactive on the labour market (including people who are retired, disabled, or fulltime housekeeping).

Second, we use a variable for occupational prestige. Questions that measure the respondents' profession were also asked to respondents who were not currently in employment but had worked in the past. Because the occupational prestige of these respondents is also relevant, especially considering life satisfaction, we also take their occupational prestige into account. We have recoded the respondents' profession into the International Socio-Economic Index (ISEI), which is an internationally comparable measure of occupational prestige (Ganzeboom et al. 1992). ISEI scores represent a continuous approach to occupational stratification and reflect a weighted sum of the average education and average income of occupational groups (Ganzeboom et al. 1992). In our sample, the ISEI scores range from 19 to 90. We include a dummy variable which indicates that for part of the respondents, about 9 %, the occupational prestige measure was not available. This method is to be preferred over removing such a large portion of respondents by listwise deletion. Respondents with missing information on occupational prestige were given the mean score on occupational prestige, which means that this group does not influence the effect of occupational prestige in our models.

Third, we use a variable for household income. The European Social Survey uses a decile approach to income, meaning that respondents are placed in ten equal income categories within the income distribution of their own country. This results in a variable with scores from one to ten, with a score of one meaning that a respondent finds his or her household income in the bottom 10 % of the national income distribution. As is often the case in survey research, quite some respondents have refused to answer the question on their income. Moreover, income data was unavailable for the respondents from Portugal. Therefore, we have created a dummy variable indicating whether income information was missing, which applies to about 24 % of the respondents. These respondents were given the mean score on household income, which means that this group does not influence the effect of household income in our analysis.

Furthermore, we use two subjective indicators of economic position, job satisfaction and experienced financial difficulties. Regarding job satisfaction, respondents were asked: 'How satisfied are you in your main job?'. Respondents could answer on an 11-point scale ranging from 0 (extremely dissatisfied) to 10 (extremely satisfied). Regarding financial difficulties, respondents were asked: 'Which of these descriptions comes closest to how you feel about your household's income nowadays?', to which respondents could answer (1) 'Living comfortably on present income', (2) 'Coping on present income', (3) 'Finding it difficult on present income', or (4) 'Finding it very difficult on present income'. We have recoded this measure as a dichotomous variable, with the first category indicating that respondents do not experience any financial difficulties (0) and the other category indicating that respondents have to do their best (cope) or even find it difficult to make ends meet (1).

Regarding perceived discrimination, respondents were asked 'Would you describe yourself as being a member of a group that is discriminated against in this country?', to which respondents could answer 'yes' or 'no'. This results in a

Table 5.1 Descriptive statistics of life satisfaction, happiness and independent variables

		Majority N = 35,383		Ethnic minority N = 1,586	
	Range	Mean/proportion[a]	SD	Mean/proportion[a]	SD
Dependent variable					
Life satisfaction	0–10	6.97	2.18	6.50	2.44
Happiness	0–10	7.25	1.92	6.99	2.14
Economic position					
Employment status					
Employed	0/1	.48		.49	
Student	0/1	.09		.10	
Unemployed	0/1	.05		.08	
Inactive	0/1	.39		.33	
Occupational prestige	19–90	44.42	13.93	42.66	13.38
Occupational prestige missing	0/1	.09		.13	
Household income	1–10	5.31	2.42	4.77	2.39
Household income missing	0–1	.24		.22	
Economic experience					
Job satisfaction	0–10	7.42	1.30	7.26	1.51
Financial difficulties	0/1	.71		.81	
Discrimination					
Perceived discrimination	0/1	.05		.32	
Individual level control variables					
Female	0/1	.53		.52	
Age	14–101	48.63	18.61	42.13	16.90
Education	0–6	2.63	1.85	2.67	1.95
Country level control variables					
Population size	1.34–81.78	22.98	25.61	22.31	26.30
Unemployment rate	3.50–20.10	9.78	4.00	10.35	4.41
Social expenditures	13.00–28.40	21.52	3.83	20.31	4.30

Source: Own calculations (ESS 5)
[a]Proportions are reported for dichotomous variables

dummy variable indicating whether respondents perceive discrimination (1) or not (0).

We use three individual level control variables in the analysis; age, gender and educational level. The variable for education has seven categories that are based on the ISCED classification of education used in the European Social Survey. We also include three country level control variables, namely the population size, the unemployment rate, and social expenditure (in percentage of GDP, based on figures from 2007). Table 5.1 shows the descriptive statistics for all variables included in our analysis.

Methods

First, it could be argued that the more subjective measures that we use of economic position and discrimination (job satisfaction, financial difficulties and the measure of perceived discrimination) are conceptually and may be empirically quite closely related to subjective well-being. Therefore, it should be noted that we have first explored the extent of endogeneity of these factors with subjective well-being by inspecting the bivariate correlations. The analysis shows that the two dependent variables, life satisfaction and happiness, are highly correlated (Pearson's $r = .72$). The bivariate correlations between life satisfaction and happiness, on the one hand, and job satisfaction, financial difficulties and perceived discrimination, on the other, are much lower. Regarding financial difficulties these correlations are highest, though only moderate in strength (Pearson's r with life satisfaction $= -.43$; with happiness $= -.39$). Regarding job satisfaction they are lower (Pearson's r with life satisfaction $= .24$; with happiness $= .22$), and regarding perceived discrimination they are lowest (Pearson's r with life satisfaction $= -.10$; with happiness $= -.08$) also among the subsample of ethnic minorities (Pearson's r with life satisfaction $= -.17$; with happiness $= -.16$). While some element of endogeneity is almost inevitable, the bivariate correlations thus suggest that this does not invalidate the current research design.

For our main analysis, we have estimated multilevel regression models with the 'xtmixed' procedure in STATA 12. This method allows simultaneous modelling of the effects of the country-level and individual-level independent variables (Hox 2002; Snijders and Bosker 1999). With multilevel modelling, variance explained by factors at the country level and variance explained by factors at the individual level can be distinguished and standard errors are estimated correctly. We have centred the independent variables on the overall mean because we also include interactions in our models. Furthermore, we have applied the design weights provided in the ESS data, which correct for country differences in sampling.

Results

The descriptive statistics in Table 5.1 already suggest that subjective well-being is indeed lower among ethnic minority members than among majority members. T-tests indicate that the group differences in observed mean scores in life satisfaction ($t(36{,}967) = 8.345$, $p < .001$) and happiness ($t(36{,}967) = 5.248$, $p < .001$) are significant. Furthermore, the differences in the indicators for economic position and perceived discrimination are also in the expected direction. It can be observed in Table 5.1 that ethnic minority members are on average more often unemployed, have lower occupational prestige scores, lower household income, lower job satisfaction, more financial difficulties, and that they perceive more discrimination.

The descriptive results therefore warrant further testing of our hypotheses with multilevel regression models.

Multilevel Analysis of Life Satisfaction

When we estimate an 'empty model' for life satisfaction, without including explanatory variables, we can see that the individual level variance (4.181) is substantially larger than the variance at the country level (.640). Though country level factors are of course important, this suggests that there is more variation in life satisfaction within countries than there is between countries in Europe.

Turning to the results presented in Table 5.2, the first model confirms that there is a significant difference in life satisfaction between people who identify as a member of an ethnic minority group and those who consider themselves part of the majority population, also when we take into account the individual and country level control variables. Model 2 in Table 5.2 shows that the difference between minority members and majority members becomes smaller when we introduce the objective economic indicators to the model, but the difference remains significant. In the third model of Table 5.2, the difference between minority members and majority members is again reduced, now by including the subjective economic indicators in the model, but the difference still remains significant. Finally, in the fourth model of Table 5.2, we include perceived discrimination and in this model the difference between ethnic minority and majority members is reduced to non-significance. This means that the differences in perceived discrimination and economic position between ethnic minority and majority members together fully mediate, in other words explain, the group differences in life satisfaction.

Looking at the final model of Table 5.2, we see that both economic position and perceived discrimination are related to life satisfaction, while self-identification as a member of an ethnic minority group is not. The model shows that life satisfaction is higher among students and lower among the unemployed, compared to respondents in paid employment. Furthermore, occupational prestige, household income and job satisfaction are shown to be positively related to life satisfaction, while experiencing financial difficulties and discrimination is associated with lower life satisfaction. Regarding the control variables, we find that both the individual level variables and the country level variables are not significantly associated with life satisfaction.

Multilevel Analysis of Happiness

An 'empty model' for happiness, which does not include any explanatory variables, shows that the individual level variance (3.348) is much larger than the variance at

Table 5.2 Multilevel regression analysis of life satisfaction

	M1: + origin group			M2: + economic position			M3: + economic experience			M4: + discrimination		
	b	se	p	b	se	p	b	se	p	b	se	p
Origin group												
(Majority = ref.)	–			–			–			–		
Ethnic minority	–.466	.106	***	–.324	.101	**	–.268	.100	**	–.086	.091	
Economic position												
Employment status												
(Employed = ref.)				–			–			–		
Student				.600	.086	***	.502	.071	***	.497	.073	***
Unemployed				–.810	.093	***	–.812	.087	***	–.794	.089	***
Inactive				–.023	.038		–.021	.043		–.010	.043	
Occupational prestige				.006	.002	***	.003	.002	*	.003	.002	*
Occupational prestige missing				.143	.049	**	.099	.045	*	.094	.047	*
Household income				.139	.014	***	.091	.014	***	.088	.014	***
Household income missing				.079	.052		.086	.050		.083	.050	
Economic experience												
Job satisfaction							.279	.010	***	.275	.010	***
Financial difficulties							–.652	.053	***	–.637	.052	***
Discrimination												
Perceived discrimination										–.697	.087	***
Individual control variables												
Female	.024	.031		.048	.034		.055	.033		.054	.033	
Age	–.007	.002	**	.000	.003		–.002	.002		–.003	.002	
Education	.094	.016	***	.031	.014	*	.008	.012		.025	.014	

Country control variables												
Population size	−.003	.005		−.002	.005		−.001	.004		−.002	.004	
Unemployment rate	−.084	.049		−.080	.048		−.062	.038		−.063	.038	
Social expenditures	.027	.039		.024	.037		.011	.031		.012	.031	
Intercept	7.423	1.090	***	6.205	1.020	***	5.202	.846	***	5.264	.847	***
N		36,969			36,969			36,969			36,969	
−2*Log Likelihood		156,964			155,215			153,168			152,915	
Δ -2*Log Likelihood (df)		948	(7)		1,749	(7)		2,047	(2)		253	(1)
Variance components												
Individual level variance		4.076			3.888			3.679			3.654	
% explained		2.5			7.0			12.0			12.6	
Country level variance		.424			.400			.275			.278	
% explained		33.8			37.5			57.0			56.7	

Source: Own calculations (ESS 5)
The relation is statistically significant at *** $p < .001$, ** $p < .01$, * $p < .05$
Note: One-tailed test for hypothesized effects

the country level (.387). Like with life satisfaction, this suggests that there is more variation in happiness within countries than there is between countries in Europe.

Regarding the results presented in Table 5.3, Model 1 confirms that there is a significant difference in happiness between people who identify as a member of an ethnic minority group and members of the majority population, when taking into account the effects of the individual and country level control variables. Model 2 in Table 5.2 shows that this difference between minority members and majority members already becomes smaller when we include the objective economic indicators in the analysis, but the variable for ethnic minority membership remains significant. In the third model of Table 5.2, the difference between minority members and majority members is further reduced by introducing the subjective economic indicators to the model.

When we include perceived discrimination in the fourth model of Table 5.3, the association between ethnic minority membership and happiness is reduced to about zero, actually even being slightly positive instead of negative. This means that the differences in happiness between ethnic minority and majority members can be fully explained by the group differences in economic position and perceived discrimination. Taking together the findings on life satisfaction and happiness, we thus find support for our first and second hypothesis.

Looking at the final model of Table 5.3, we see that both economic position and perceived discrimination are related to happiness. The model shows that happiness is higher among students and lower among the unemployed, compared to respondents in paid employment. Furthermore, occupational prestige, household income and job satisfaction are shown to be positively related to happiness, while experiencing financial difficulties and discrimination is associated with lower life satisfaction. Regarding the control variables, happiness is higher among women, among younger respondents and among the higher educated, while the country level control variables are not significantly associated with happiness.

Interaction Effects

Tables 5.2 and 5.3 have only clarified the main effects of minority group status and the other hypothesized correlates of life satisfaction and happiness. However, it could also be that the economic factors, such as household income, or perceived discrimination, are differently related to subjective well-being among majority members than among those who self-identify as member of an ethnic minority group. To investigate this possibility, we turn to the results of a test of interaction effects presented in Table 5.4. All the interaction effects in Table 5.4 were tested in separate models that also control for the variables included in the final models of Tables 5.2 and 5.3. In case the interaction effects show up to be significant, this means that for instance perceived discrimination has a different impact on life satisfaction or happiness among the majority population than it does among ethnic minority group members.

Table 5.3 Multilevel regression analysis of happiness

	M1: + origin group			M2: + economic position			M3: + economic experience			M4: + discrimination		
	b	se	p	b	se	p	b	se	p	b	se	p
Origin group												
(Majority = ref.)	–			–			–			–		
Ethnic minority	–.258	.061	***	–.143	.055	**	–.101	.056	*	.038	.051	
Economic position												
Employment status												
(Employed = ref.)				–			–			–		
Student				.400	.074	***	.332	.063	***	.327	.063	***
Unemployed				–.620	.095	***	–.631	.099	***	–.618	.101	***
Inactive				–.013	.031		–.012	.032		–.004	.032	
Occupational prestige				.004	.001	**	.002	.001		.002	.001	*
Occupational prestige missing				.007	.061		–.029	.060		–.033	.061	
Household income				.117	.011	***	.083	.012	***	.081	.012	***
Household income missing				.052	.041		.059	.041		.057	.041	
Economic experience												
Job satisfaction							.240	.013	***	.237	.013	***
Financial difficulties							–.429	.037	***	–.418	.036	***
Discrimination												
Perceived discrimination										–.534	.070	***
Individual control variables												
Female	.049	.033		.076	.035	*	.080	.035	*	.079	.035	*
Age	–.009	.002	***	–.004	.002		–.006	.002	**	–.007	.002	**
Education	.087	.016	***	.031	.014	*	.027	.014		.027	.014	*

(continued)

Table 5.3 (continued)

	M1: + origin group			M2: + economic position			M3: + economic experience			M4: + discrimination		
	b	se	p	b	se	p	b	se	p	b	se	p
Country control variables												
Population size	−.001	.004		−.001	.003		−.000	.003		−.000	.003	
Unemployment rate	−.059	.038		−.056	.037		−.043	.029		−.044	.029	
Social expenditures	.033	.027		.030	.025		.021	.021		.022	.021	
Intercept	7.400	.774	***	6.500	.740	***	5.470	.604	***	5.518	.603	***
N		36,969			36,969			36,969			36,969	
−2*Log Likelihood		148,162			146,837			145,218			145,034	
Δ -2*Log Likelihood (df)		1,506	(7)		1,325	(7)		1,619	(2)		184	(1)
Variance components												
Individual level variance		3.213			3.100			2.968			2.953	
% explained		4.0			7.4			11.3			11.7	
Country level variance		.243			.227			.156			.157	
% explained		37.2			41.3			59.7			59.4	

Source: Own calculations (ESS 5)

The relation is statistically significant at *** $p < .001$, ** $p < .01$, * $p < .05$

Note: One-tailed test for hypothesized effects

Looking at the first column of Table 5.4, it becomes clear that the effects of economic position and perceived discrimination differ very little between ethnic minority and majority group members. Regarding life satisfaction, only the interactions between ethnic minority membership and being unemployed and between ethnic minority membership and economic inactivity are significant. This means that unemployment and economic inactivity more strongly depress life satisfaction

Table 5.4 Final models (Model 4, Tables 5.2 and 5.3) + interactions, N = 36,969

	Life Satisfaction								
	Interaction effect			Simple slope among majority			Simple slope among ethnic minority		
	b	se	p	b	se	p	b	se	p
Economic position									
x Student	−.173	.247		.501	.073	***	.328	.249	
x Unemployed	**−.564**	**.283**	*	**−.758**	**.097**	***	**−1.322**	**.246**	***
x Inactive	**−.309**	**.148**	*	**.003**	**.045**		**−.305**	**.141**	*
x Occupational prestige	.002	.005		.003	.002		.005	.005	
x Household income	.010	.028		.088	.014	***	.098	.031	**
Economic experience									
x Job satisfaction	−.051	.047		.278	.011	***	.228	.041	***
x Financial difficulties	−.140	.136		−.632	.051	***	−.773	.151	***
Discrimination									
x Perceived discrimination	.172	.139		−.729	.084	***	−.556	.160	***
	Happiness								
	Interaction effect			Simple slope among majority			Simple slope among ethnic minority		
	b	se	p	b	se	p	b	se	p
Economic position									
x Student	−.284	.213		.338	.067	***	.054	.200	
x Unemployed	−.202	.133		−.607	.107	***	−.810	.105	***
x Inactive	**−.307**	**.128**	*	**.010**	**.032**		**−.297**	**.128**	*
x Occupational prestige	−.000	.005		.002	.001		.002	.005	
x Household income	.024	.023		.080	.012	***	.103	.026	***
Economic experience									
x Job satisfaction	.020	.035		.236	.013	***	.256	.033	***
x Financial difficulties	.040	.112		−.420	.037	***	−.380	.101	***
Discrimination									
x Perceived discrimination	.047	.102		−.543	.070	***	−.496	.116	***

Source: Own calculations (ESS 5)
The relation is statistically significant at *** $p < .001$, ** $p < .01$, * $p < .05$
Note: Significant interaction effects and respective simple slopes in bold print. All interaction effects were tested separately in models that further include all the variables of the final model (Model 4 of Tables 5.2 and 5.3). Full models available from the authors

among minority groups than among the majority population. Regarding happiness, only the interaction between minority group membership and being inactive on the labour market is significant. For all other indicators of economic position, and regarding perceived discrimination, the association with subjective well-being is the same for majority group members and ethnic minority members.

The interaction effect between ethnic minority membership and being unemployed, regarding life satisfaction, modestly goes in the direction of our third hypothesis. This becomes clear from the results in the second and third column of Table 5.4, which show that the simple slopes for the effect of being unemployed are negative for both groups, but the estimate is larger for ethnic minority members. Concerning the significant interactions between minority group membership and economic inactivity, regarding both life satisfaction and happiness, the simple slopes indicate that the effect of being inactive is about zero for majority members and negative for ethnic minority members, which is consistent with our third hypothesis. All in all however, we find limited support for our hypothesis that economic position and perceived discrimination are more strongly related to subjective well-being among ethnic minority members than among members of the majority.

Discussion

Our study confirms the expectation that subjective well-being, in terms of life satisfaction and happiness, is lower among people who self-identify as a member of an ethnic minority group compared to those who consider themselves to be part of the majority population. The most important conclusion, however, is that these differences can be fully explained by the fact that ethnic minority members occupy more disadvantaged socio-economic positions in European societies and experience more discrimination. This is an important addition to previous studies among immigrant populations in Europe, which have concluded that levels of life satisfaction among immigrants are lower than among the majority population and which have suggested explanations for these differences (De Vroome and Hooghe 2013; Safi 2010). Where these previous studies emphasized the disadvantage in life satisfaction of minorities that are externally classified as first or second generation immigrant, our study adds that the qualitatively different group of people who self-identify as a member of an ethnic minority group are faced with a similar disadvantage.

Moreover, our results at first sight contrast the results of previous research among immigrant populations in Europe. Safi (2010) concludes, on the basis of a cross-national study in European countries, that a difference between native majority populations and first and second generation immigrant groups remains after controlling for important correlates of life satisfaction, including perceived discrimination, which is shown to be a consistent predictor of life satisfaction. Though we focus on a different type of minority group, close inspection of our results is actually in line with the interpretation that discrimination is perhaps the most crucial explanatory factor with regard to the subjective well-being of minority groups in society. The differences in subjective well-being between majority group members and minority group members are fully explained when we take into account both perceived discrimination and a broad set of indicators of economic position, and behind the disadvantaged economic position of the ethnic minority groups in our study may very well lie processes of structural discrimination.

In any case, our study provides strong support for a need-gratification theory of subjective well-being. In line with this theoretical perspective, our study shows that adverse living conditions among ethnic minority populations lead to differences in subjective well-being between majority and ethnic minority groups, as both economic positions and discrimination can be related to universal needs for safety, belonging, esteem and self-actualization. Our study therefore adds further support to macro-level country comparisons and national studies that have previously found support for a need-gratification approach to subjective well-being (de Vroome and Hooghe 2013; Oishi et al. 1999; Veenhoven 1991). Furthermore, the fact that we find only few significant interaction effects suggests that the explanatory factors derived from need-gratification theory apply equally well to very diverse groups in European societies, in this case ethnic minority members and majority group members. In addition to need-gratification theory and the related role of discrimination, our results also seem to be in line with a social comparison theory of subjective well-being, as the lower consumption levels and loss of status that are associated with income and financial difficulties play an important role (Guillen-Royo 2008). We would therefore conclude that these theoretical approaches to subjective well-being are largely complementary.

From a policy perspective, it is important to note that levels of life satisfaction and happiness are not inevitably lower among ethnic minority populations than among majority populations. With specific policies aiming to reduce prejudice and structural discrimination, steps can be taken to improve the living conditions of ethnic minority populations. Our results indicate that these steps are necessary if policy makers would want to achieve equal levels of quality of life among diverse population groups. Because a sense of relative deprivation among ethnic minority groups can be associated with socially disruptive behaviour, such as criminality and radicalism, the perspective that inequalities in subjective well-being between social groups can feasibly be reduced to zero should be encouraging.

A remarkable finding is that the relation between perceived discrimination and subjective well-being is similar for minority and majority group members. We had actually hypothesized that the negative effect of perceived discrimination would be stronger among minority group members, as a sense of collective identity and self-esteem is likely more salient among these groups. Though it goes beyond the scope of our present analysis, perhaps the role of social identity processes should be considered more extensively in future studies on differences in subjective well-being between population groups, as the literature further suggests that ethnic identification can also have a positive impact on subjective well-being among minority groups (Kennedy and Cummins 2007; Verkuyten 2008). Relatedly, it is possible that the relatively strong social networks within minority communities have a positive impact, which could contrast with the community spirit among members of the general population that is sometimes thought to be declining (Putnam 2000).

We also want to mention some limitations to the present study. First, it has to be noted that the more subjective measures of economic position and the measure of perceived discrimination may be endogenous to subjective well-being to some extent. Analysis shows that the bivariate correlations between these factors and the measures of happiness and life satisfaction are not that strong, however, suggesting that they are clearly independent constructs rather than alternative indicators for subjective well-being. Therefore, the level of endogeneity in these measures, which is to some extent inevitable with subjective indicators, does not seem to invalidate our research design. Second, because the data we use here is cross-sectional, they do not allow us to test in a strict manner the causality of the proposed relations. However, our explanations are theoretically derived, and regarding perceived discrimination the reverse causal order is much less logical. Regarding economic position, the possible impact on subjective well-being is also well-established in the literature, though a bidirectional relationship remains possible.

Appendix

Table A.1 Cross-classification of externally defined migration status and self-classification as majority or ethnic minority group member

	Self-defined classification		
Immigration status	Majority	Ethnic minority	Total
Native	**30,891**	**484**	**31,375**
% within self-defined classification	87.4 %	30.7 %	84.9 %
First generation immigrant	**2,338**	**850**	**3,188**
% within self-defined classification	6.6 %	53.8 %	8.6 %
Second generation immigrant	**2,134**	**245**	**2,379**
% within Minority group	6.0 %	15.5 %	6.4 %
Total	**35,363**	**1,579**	**36,942**
% within self-defined classification	100.0 %	100.0 %	100.0 %

Note: The total N (39,942) is slightly lower than in the main analysis, due to missing information on immigration status

References

Ahmed, P., Feliciano, C., & Emigh, R. J. (2007). Internal and external ethnic assessments in Eastern Europe. *Social Forces, 86*, 231–255.

Angner, E. (2010). Subjective well-being. *The Journal of Socio-Economics, 39*, 361–368.

Anthias, F. (2001). The concept of 'social division' and theorising social stratification: Looking at ethnicity and class. *Sociology, 35*, 835–854.

Bălţătescu, S. (2007). Central and Eastern Europeans migrants' subjective quality of life: A comparative study. *Journal of Identity and Migration Studies, 1*, 67–81.

Bartram, D. (2011). Economic migration and happiness: Comparing immigrants' and natives' happiness gains from income. *Social Indicators Research, 103*, 57–76.

Branscombe, N. R., Schmitt, M. T., & Harvey, R. D. (1999). Perceiving pervasive discrimination among African Americans: Implications for group identification and well-being. *Journal of Personality and Social Psychology, 77*, 135–149.

Cassidy, C., O'Connor, R. C., Howe, C., & Warden, D. (2004). Perceived discrimination and psychological distress: The role of personal and ethnic self-esteem. *Journal of Counseling Psychology, 51*, 329–339.

Cheung, C., & Leung, K. (2004). Forming life satisfaction among different social groups during the modernization of China. *Journal of Happiness Studies, 5*, 23–56.

Cooper, H. (2002). Investigating socio-economic explanations for gender and ethnic inequalities in health. *Social Science & Medicine, 54*, 693–706.

De Jong, G. F., & Madamba, A. B. (2001). A double disadvantage? Minority group, immigrant status, and underemployment in the United States. *Social Science Quarterly, 82*, 117–130.

De Vroome, T., & Hooghe, M. (2013). Life satisfaction among ethnic minorities in the Netherlands: Immigration experience or adverse living conditions? *Journal of Happiness Studies*. doi:10.1007/s10902-013-9483-2.

Diener, E. (2000). Subjective well-being. The science of happiness and a proposal for a national index. *American Psychologist, 55*, 34–43.

Diener, E., & Diener, M. (1995). Cross-cultural correlates of life satisfaction and self-esteem. *Journal of Personality and Social Psychology, 68*, 653–663.

Ganzeboom, H. B. G., De Graaf, P. M., & Treiman, D. J. (1992). A standard international socio-economic index of occupational status. *Social Science Research, 21*, 1–56.

Guillen-Royo, M. (2008). Consumption and subjective wellbeing: Exploring basic needs, social comparison, social integration and hedonism in Peru. *Social Indicators Research, 89*, 535–555.

Heady, B., Muffels, R., & Wooden, M. (2004). *Money doesn't buy happiness.... Or does it? A reconsideration based on the combined effects of wealth, income and consumption* (IZA Discussion Paper No. 1218). http://ssrn.com/abstract=571661. Accessed 17 July 2012.

Hox, J. (2002). *Multilevel analysis. Techniques and applications*. Mahwah: Erlbaum.

Jasinskaja-Lahti, I., Liebkind, K., & Solheim, E. (2009). To identify or not to identify? National disidentification as an alternative reaction to perceived ethnic discrimination. *Applied Psychology: An International Review, 58*, 105–128.

Kennedy, W. L., & Cummins, R. A. (2007). Ethnic identity and subjective wellbeing: Connections and possibilities. *The International Journal of Diversity in Organizations, Communities and Nations, 7*, 107–116.

Lenski, G. (1966). *Power in privilege: A theory of social stratification*. New York: McGraw-Hill.

Maslow, A. H. (1970). *Motivation and personality*. New York: Harper & Row.

Moghaddam, M. (2008). Happiness, faith, friends, and fortune: Empirical evidence from the 1998 US survey data. *Journal of Happiness Studies, 9*, 577–587.

Nazroo, J. Y. (2003). The structuring of ethnic inequalities in health: Economic position, racial discrimination, and racism. *American Journal of Public Health, 93*, 277–284.

Oishi, S., Diener, E. F., Lucas, R. E., & Suh, E. M. (1999). Cross-cultural variations in predictors of life satisfaction: Perspectives from needs and values. *Personality and Social Psychology Bulletin, 25*, 980–990.

Olgiati, A., Calvo, R., & Berkman, L. (2013). Are migrants going up a blind alley? Economic migration and life satisfaction around the world: Cross-national evidence from Europe, North America, and Australia. *Social Indicators Research, 114*, 383–404.

Putnam, R. (2000). *Bowling alone*. New York: Simon & Schuster.

Rooth, D., & Ekberg, J. (2003). Unemployment and earnings for second generation immigrants in Sweden. Ethnic background and parent composition. *Journal of Population Economics, 16*, 787–814.

Safi, M. (2010). Immigrants' life satisfaction in Europe: Between assimilation and discrimination. *European Sociological Review, 26*, 159–176.

Slack, T., & Jensen, L. (2002). Race, ethnicity, and underemployment in nonmetropolitan America: A 30-year profile. *Rural Sociology, 67*, 208–233.

Snijders, T., & Bosker, R. (1999). *Multilevel analysis*. London: Sage.

Thomassen, B. (2010). 'Second generation immigrants' or 'Italians with immigrant parents'? Italian and European perspectives on immigrants and their children. *Bulletin of Italian Politics, 2*, 21–44.

Utsey, S. O., Chae, M. H., Brown, C. F., & Kelly, D. (2002). Effect of ethnic group membership on ethnic identity, race-related stress and quality of life. *Cultural Diversity and Ethnic Minority Psychology, 8*, 366–377.

Van Tubergen, F. (2006). *Immigrant integration: A cross-national study*. New York: LFB Scholarly Publishing LLC.

Veenhoven, R. (1991). Is happiness relative? *Social Indicators Research, 24*, 1–34.

Veenhoven, R. (2004). Happiness as a public policy aim: The greatest happiness principle. In A. Linley & S. Joseph (Eds.), *Positive psychology in practice* (pp. 658–678). Hoboken: Wiley.

Verkuyten, M. (2008). Life satisfaction among ethnic minorities: The role of discrimination and group identification. *Social Indicators Research, 89*, 391–404.

Vohra, N., & Adair, J. (2000). Life satisfaction of Indian immigrants in Canada. *Psychology & Developing Societies, 12*, 109–138.

Williams, D. R., Neighbors, H. W., & Jackson, J. S. (2003). Racial/ethnic discrimination and health: Findings from community studies. *American Journal of Public Health, 93*, 200–208.

Zick, A., Pettigrew, T. F., & Wagner, U. (2008). Ethnic prejudice and discrimination in Europe. *Journal of Social Issues, 64*, 233–251.

Chapter 6
Self-Evaluation Affects Subjective Well-Being: The Effects of Socioeconomic Status and Personality in Taiwan

Hsiu-Jen Yeh, Yeu-Sheng Hsieh, and Ruey-Ming Tsay

Introduction

There is a large literature on quality of life in western industrialized countries, but relatively few researchers in Taiwan have addressed the topic (Tsou and Liu 2001; Tsai 2007, 2009; Tsai et al. 2012; Liao et al. 2005; Lu et al. 2011; Chang 2011; Chang 2013; Yeh 2015). According to Veenhoven (2000), quality of life can be classified as two axes—the combination of life chances (determinants of quality of life) and life outcomes (degree of quality of life), and four dimensions of the outer and inner aspects of quality of life—(1) the livability of an environment (outer quality of life chances), including material conditions and social characteristics; (2) life-ability (inner quality of life chances) which also entails psychological capital, including the power or efficacy associated with the potential to cope with adversaries; (3) life utility (outer quality of life outcomes), which refers to transcendental quality of life concepts or ultimate meanings that go beyond one's subjective perceptions; and (4) life appreciation (inner quality of life outcomes), referring to the subjective evaluation of one's own life, also described as subjective well-being (SWB), life satisfaction, or happiness. The fourth dimension is the most frequently studied.

In this study we will focus on the three quality of life dimensions, namely, relationships among environmental livability (outer quality of life chances), measured as socioeconomic status (SES), including absolute and relative income and

H.-J. Yeh (✉)
Department of Social Welfare, National Chung Cheng University,
168 University Road, Chia-Yi 62102, Taiwan
e-mail: hjjyeh@gmail.com

Y.-S. Hsieh
Department of Bio-Industry Communication and Development,
National Taiwan University, Taipei, Taiwan

R.-M. Tsay
Department of Sociology, Tunghai University, Taichung, Taiwan

F. Maggino (ed.), *A New Research Agenda for Improvements in Quality of Life*,
Social Indicators Research Series 57, DOI 10.1007/978-3-319-15904-1_6

objective and subjective class; life-ability (inner quality of life chances), measured in terms of Big Five personality traits, and appreciation of life (inner quality of life outcomes), measured as subjective well-being, including life satisfaction and happiness. Further, we examine the relative effects of socioeconomic status and personality on subjective well-being in Taiwan. Whereas the majority of studies on the effect of socioeconomic status on well-being focuses on income only, we use a sociological perspective to expand the scope of SES to include absolute and relative income as well as objective and subjective class position. This article uses life satisfaction and happiness to measure subjective well-being as most well-being research did, since past research have shown that life satisfaction and happiness each captures different dimensions of subjective well-being. Although life satisfaction and happiness, as the two measures of SWB, tend to be positively related, this study considers it is more appropriate to analyze them separately.

Based on the substantial body of research on the relationship between socioeconomic status and subjective well-being, especially in terms of income (Cummins 2000; Gitmez and Morcöl 1994; Dolan et al. 2008), the present study asks the following three questions: (a) What mechanism explains the relationship between two types of income, absolute and relative, and subjective well-being in Taiwan, and which one is relatively important? (b) How do objective and subjective class positions affect SWB in Taiwan, and what is their relative importance? (c) After accounting for SES in terms of income and class, does personality still exert an independent effect on SWB in Taiwan, and what is the relative importance of SES and personality traits? We will argue that even though absolute SES exerts a positive effect on individual well-being, it is relative SES that plays a more important role. Further, after accounting for the effects of absolute and relative SES, it is positive personality traits that determine how well an individual evaluates his or her well-being.

This study makes four major contributions to the research of well-being. First, past research that investigated the link between socioeconomic status and well-being are mostly based on an economic approach that emphasizes only on income, either in terms of absolute income or relative income. Using a sociological approach, this study highlights the importance of class position to well-being, and includes income and class dimensions of SES into the analysis of well-being. Second, compared to previous research, we use better refined measures of SES in terms of absolute and relative income as well as objective and subjective class position. Third, our analytical results indicate independent effect of class position (especially subjective class position) on well-being, which strongly justifies the importance of class dimension, in addition to income, on well-being research. Fourth, we are perhaps the first study that has simultaneously examined the effect of SES and personality traits on well-being in Taiwan.

Theoretical Framework and Hypotheses

To date, research on well-being has been dominated by economists and psychologists, but the past decade has witnessed an increase in sociological research focusing on happiness trends in terms of age, cohort, and period dimensions (Yang 2008), on familial and psychological origins of happiness (Schnittker 2008), on the effects of neighborhood on well-being (Firebaugh and Schroeder 2009; Hou 2014), and on the relationship between well-being and religion (Hout and Greeley 2012). However, the literature is still dominated by two approaches. Economics-focused researchers argue that a society's average consumption level increases as average income level increases, and when the basic needs of individuals are satisfied as income increases, their well-being consequently increases. In contrast, psychology-focused researchers emphasize the importance of personality traits on subjective well-being, and argue that income level is not a necessary condition for SWB.

Four major theories have been established to explain the relationship between socioeconomic status and subjective well-being.

1. Absolute Theory. This theory emphasizes the importance of basic needs in increasing a sense of well-being. For example, Okulicz-Kozaryn (2011), using General Social Survey, found that net of the effect of age, sex, marital status, health status, occupation, and working hours, absolute family income exerts a significant and positive effect on happiness in the U.S. However, Veenhoven (1988) found that when income level exceeds a threshold or absolute benchmark, the effect of income becomes much weaker. According to this theory, our first hypothesis is established as

Hypothesis 1: Absolute personal or family income exerts a positive effect on individual well-being.

2. Relative Theory. Adherents of this theory contend that the effect of income on subjective well-being depends on two factors—social comparison and individual expectations (Easterlin 1974). In other words, regardless of the size of one's income, well-being is determined by the relative position of that income and the wealth gap between the individual and a reference group (Meadow et al. 1992; Diener and Diener 1996; Parducci 1982; Clark et al. 2008; Luttmer 2005). That relative position is the essence of the Easterlin paradox, which states that happiness and income are not related after a certain point (Easterlin 1974, 1995, 2001). A variation of this theory is Durayappah's (2011) 3P Theory, a psychological theory that compares the well-being of individuals (as opposed to the well-being of reference groups) at present, past, and prospective life stages, based on their self-evaluations. The foundation for much of the work in the area of Relative Theory can be traced to Thorstein Veblen's (1899) *Theory of the Leisure Class*, and later work by the economics work of James Duesenberry (1949) on the relevance of income and consumer behavior. Veblen's "status effects" posits that one's status can be diminished by peer group status, and that relative success (social comparison)

matters most to one's well-being. Much later, Easterlin (1974, 1995, 2001) triggered a large number of studies by combining Veblen's ideas with the concepts of social comparison and adaptation (see, for example, Akerlof 1997; Oswald 1997; Clark et al. 2008; Fuentes and Rojas 2001), thereby emphasizing the effects of relative versus absolute income, the role of reference groups, relative deprivation, and concern for social status on individual well-being.

According to Akerlof and Kranton's (2000, 2010) Identity Theory, an individual's desire for superiority and concern for status are shaped by social contexts and social norms. Accordingly, relative income evaluated in terms of social comparison generates a positional identity that satisfies one's concerns for social status and sense of superiority via community approval and disapproval mechanisms. Thus, an individual's increase in relative income can be interpreted by both the individual and community as an indicator of self-enhancement or upward mobility, with the gain in positional identity increasing her subjective well-being. The converse is also true: a decrease in relative income can threaten one's self image and positional identity, thereby decreasing her subjective well-being—an example of the "envy effect" of social comparison (Brennan 1973; Frank 1985).

3. Aspiration Theory. According to this theory, life satisfaction depends on the ratio of satisfied desires to total desires. Accordingly, an individual whose desires have been satisfied will be happier than an individual with unsatisfied desires, regardless of income level; the theory assumes a strong association between income and total desires. Similar to Relative Theory, Aspiration Theory also emphasizes the role of expectation in the relationship between income level and well-being.

According to the above background, the next two hypotheses are expressed as

Hypothesis 2A: Relative personal or family income exerts positive influences on individual well-being.

Hypothesis 2B: After taking into account of the effect of absolute income, relative income alone exerts a positive influence on individual well-being.

Sociologists have long emphasized the role of social context in explaining social outcomes. For example Durkheim's (1897) research on suicide spotlighted the importance of social context on individual disposition and behavior. The fact that individuals with high incomes are more likely than those with low incomes to describe themselves as very happy is perceived as evidence indicating that the social context of a comparison plays a central role in determining happiness (Firebaugh and Schroeder 2009; Hou 2014). Schnittker (2008) has put together a detailed review of sociological research emphasizing the role of social structure and social environment on an individual's psychological state, including well-being. According to House (1981), the mechanism underlying the importance of social position in changing an individual's well-being involves the effects of exposure, learning, and reinforcement embedded in one's social environment on subjective well-being. Earlier studies gathered significant evidence indicating positive associations between happiness and both achievement and assets. Specific examples include the ways that achievement in education, work, and income lead to greater happiness (Mirowsky and Ross 1986), and the correlation between occupational self-direction and positive well-being (Schooler 1984). Income exerts a positive effect because greater income supports greater consumption and fulfillment of desired courses of action. The occupation effect emphasizes social learning—for example, individuals whose jobs encourage self-direction and personal responsibility are more likely to succeed and to enjoy a greater sense of well-being (Schooler 1984). Based on this background, the next hypothesis is expressed as

Hypothesis 3: Objective class position based on occupation exerts a positive influence on individual well-being. In other words, the higher the objective class position, the higher the level of individual well-being.

Since Relative Theory asserts that higher relative income increases subjective well-being, higher subjective class position (measure in relative terms) is a likely indicator of relative success that should promote individual well-being. Accordingly, the next two hypotheses are written as

Hypothesis 4A: Subjective class position exerts a positive influence on individual well-being. In other words, the higher the subjective class position, the higher the level of individual well-being.

Hypothesis 4B: After taking into account of the effect of objective class position, subjective class position still exerts an independent and positive influence on individual well-being.

4. Adaptation Theory. According to this theory (Helson 1964), which focuses on the effects of emotional capabilities on coping with positive and negative life events, individuals with higher adaptive capabilities tend to have greater life satisfaction even when their income levels are very low (Brickman et al. 1978). Similar to Aspiration Theory, it predicts a short-lived positive effect of income growth on gains in happiness. Since an individual's expectations increase with income, adaptation results in no permanent gain in happiness when income increases—an example of Brickman and Campbell's (1971) "hedonic treadmill" effect. A similar argument is found in Lykken and Tellegen's (1996) set point theory in psychology: it is personality traits that determine subjective well-being, and positive or negative events will only exert temporary effects on well-being, since individuals will eventually adjust to life events and return to their earlier levels of happiness as before. This is also referred to as the "habituation effect" (Firebaugh and Schroeder 2009).

According to Adaptation Theory, personality traits are important to SWB in that they reflect how an individual experiences, understands, and responds to the external world; this is the mechanism that links personality to various social outcomes (Roberts 2009). The majority of positive psychology studies have addressed the link between personality and SWB (for detailed reviews, see Albuquerque et al. 2012; Ha and Kim 2013).

The five-factor model (also known as the "Big Five"), a widely used measure of personality traits in SWB research, consists of five dimensions: extraversion, agreeableness, conscientiousness, emotional stability (also referred to as neuroticism), and openness (Gosling et al. 2003; John et al. 2008). A large number of researchers have gathered evidence indicating strong associations between greater SWB and high levels of both extraversion and emotional stability (Argyle 1999; Diener and Lucas 1999; Costa and McCrae 1980; Ha and Kim 2013). However, DeNeve and Cooper (1998) found that while both traits exert significant effects on SWB, the magnitudes of those effects are relatively small. Others have reported only moderate effects of conscientiousness on SWB (DeNeve and Cooper 1998; Lucas 2008). Studies using large and representative samples have identified only moderate effects of personality traits on SWB, after taking into account relevant covariates such as trust and religiosity (Helliwell 2006). According to the above discussion, if (as Adaptation Theory predicts) subjective well-being is primarily affected by personality traits regardless of environmental factors such as SES (i.e., income and class), after controlling for the effects of SES, personality traits should exert an independent positive effect on subjective well-being. Thus, the next hypothesis is expressed as

Hypothesis 5: After taking into account the effect of SES in terms of income and class, personality traits exert an independent and positive effect on individual well-being.

Data Source and Measures

The data used in this study were drawn from a special 2009 questionnaire on social inequality of Taiwan Social Change Survey (TSCS), a large-scale, representative, face-to-face survey conducted by Academia Sinica in Taiwan (see Academia Sinica 2014 for the details of TSCS). This survey, whose questionnaire orientation is similar to that of the General Social Survey (GSS) in the U.S. (see NORC 2014 for the details of GSS), is the most frequently analyzed collection of data on social issues by social scientists in Taiwan. While prior research that examined the effect of personality traits and well-being often used convenience samples (see Dolan et al. 2008), this study has the advantage of a better dataset by using a national representative survey so that the analytical findings of the effect of SES and personality can be generalized to the general public in Taiwan. To construct our objective class position variable, we included respondents with prior work experience, whether or not they were currently employed; however, we did carefully select respondents who could provide information regarding their current or previous jobs. This study uses Stata 13 to conduct data analysis.

Dependent Variables

Our analysis included two dependent variables, the first being "On the whole how satisfied are you with the life you lead?", a six-point ordinal scale ranging from very satisfied, to satisfied, slightly satisfied, slightly unsatisfied, unsatisfied, and very unsatisfied. Because some response categories had too few observations, this study recoded life satisfaction into a four-point ordinal scale, including unsatisfied (very unsatisfied and unsatisfied), slightly unsatisfied, slightly satisfied, and satisfied (very satisfied and satisfied) in ascending order. The second dependent variable, "Taken all together, how would you say things are these days?", is a four-point ordinal scale ranging from very happy to happy, unhappy, and very unhappy. To ensure each response category has sufficient observations, this study recoded happiness into a three-point ordinal scale, including unhappy (very unhappy and unhappy), happy, and very happy in ascending order. Table 6.1 displays the operationalization and measurement of all study variables in the analysis.

Independent Variables

The explanatory variables included the following SES factors:

1. Absolute personal income—specifically, pre-tax monthly total individual income, measured according to an ordinal scale of income categories. We took a category midpoint and converted it into an interval variable, measured in increments of $ 10,000 New Taiwan (NT) dollars.
2. Absolute family income—specifically, pre-tax monthly total family income, measured according to an ordinal scale of income categories. Similar to individual income, we took a category midpoint and converted it into an interval variable, measured in increments of $ 10,000 New Taiwan (NT) dollars.
3. Relative personal income, measured in terms of responses to the survey item, "How do you compare your current income with the income you think you deserve?" In other words, this variable measures relative success in terms of the respondent's self-evaluation of achievement. Responses were recorded as one of six categories coded as 1, "much less than I deserve"; 2, "less than I deserve"; 3, "exactly as I deserve"; 4, "more than I deserve"; 5, "much more than I deserve"; and 0 "I have never worked before."
4. Relative family income: measured in terms of responses to the survey item, "On the whole, how do you compare your current family income with current family expenditures?" This variable addresses the aspiration mechanism—that is, the idea that consumption level tends to rise with income. Responses were recorded as 1, "very short of income"; 2, "short of income"; 3, "sufficient"; and 4, "very sufficient."
5. Objective class position: coded as one of five categories: upper non-manual (managerial occupations, professionals), lower non-manual (semi-professionals,

Table 6.1 Operationalization and measurement of study variables

Variables
Dependent variables
Life satisfaction
"On the whole how satisfied are you with the life you lead?"
(unsatisfied = 1, slightly unsatisfied = 2, slightly satisfied = 3, satisfied = 4).
Happiness
"Taken all together, how would you say things are these days?"
(unhappy = 1, happy = 2, very happy = 3).
Explanatory variable
Absolute personal income: Midpoint of pre-tax monthly total personal income category (interval scale in $10,000 New Taiwan dollars).
Absolute family income: Midpoint of pre-tax monthly total family income category (interval scale in $ 10,000 New Taiwan dollars).
Relative personal income: "How do you compare your current income with the income you think you deserve?" (much less than I deserve = 1; less than I deserve = 2; exactly as I deserve = 3; more than I deserve = 4; much more than I deserve = 5; I have never worked before = 0).
Relative family income: "On the whole, how do you compare your current family income with current family expenditures?" (very short of income = 1; short of income = 2; sufficient = 3; very sufficient = 4).
Objective class position: upper non-manual = 0 (managerial occupations, professionals), lower non-manual = 1 (semi-professionals, administrators, clerical), upper manual = 2 (skilled workers, craftsmen, technicians), lower manual = 3 (semi-skilled and un-skilled workers such as mechanics and machinery operators), and agricultural = 4 (farming, fishing, forestry).
Subjective class position: lower class = 0, working class = 1, lower-middle class = 2, middle class = 3, upper-middle class = 4 (including upper class).
Personality traits
Extraversion: the sum of (1) + (2), where (1) "I accomplish every day's workload even if I don't feel well" and (2) "I get things done in order to earn compliments."
Agreeableness: the sum of (3) + (4), where (3) "I get along well with others" and (4) "I am not good at dealing with conflicts" (reverse-coded).
Conscientiousness: the sum of (5) + (6), where (5) "I am very confident in getting my plan completed" and (6) "No matter what kind of job I am doing, I can do it as well as others."
Emotional stability: the sum of (7) + (8), where (7) "I can always control things that occur to me" and (8) "I have nothing to be proud of" (reverse coded).
Openness: the sum of (9) + (10), where (9) "Even if I dislike my work, I still do my best to finish it" and (10) "Even if a task takes a long time to achieve the outcome, I still keep up with it."
Control variables
Age (continuous scale in years)
Sex (men = 0, women = 1)
Education (<high school = 0, college and above = 1)
Working status (not working = 0, working = 1)
Marital status (never married = 0, divorced/separated/widowed = 1, married = 2)
Health status (healthy = 0, not healthy = 1)
Residence (urban = 0, rural = 1)
Religion (no religion = 0, yes = 1)

administrators, clerical), upper manual (skilled workers, craftsmen, technicians), lower manual (semi-skilled and un-skilled workers such as mechanics and machinery operators), and agricultural (farming, fishing, forestry).

6. Subjective class position, measured as one of six self-identified categories: upper class, upper-middle class, middle class, lower-middle class, working class, and lower class. To ensure each response category has sufficient observations, this study recoded subjective class position into a five-categories ordinal scale, including lower class, working class, lower middle class, middle class, and upper middle class (upper class and upper middle class).

Our explanatory variables also included five personality trait dimensions, each represented by the summed scores of responses to two items (four-point scale of "strongly agree," "agree," "disagree," and "strongly disagree"). The first trait, extraversion, reflects the extent to which an individual is energetic, outgoing, and positive; the second, agreeableness, reflects the extent to which an individual is warm, sympathetic, cooperative, and capable of getting along well with others; the third, conscientiousness, reflects the extent to which an individual is organized, punctual, and dependable; the fourth, emotional stability, reflects the extent to which an individual is worry-free, immune to stress, and less prone to negative affect; and the fifth, openness, reflects the extent to which an individual is open-minded, creative, and aesthetic (Funder and Fast 2010; Ha and Kim 2013).

Extraversion was measured as the sum of responses to items (1) "I accomplish every day's workload even if I don't feel well" and (2) "I get things done in order to earn compliments." Agreeableness was measured as the sum of responses to items (3) "I get along well with others" and (4) "I am not good at dealing with conflicts" (reverse-coded). Conscientiousness was measured as the sum of responses to items (5) "I am very confident in getting my plan completed" and (6) "No matter what kind of job I am doing, I can do it as well as others." Emotional stability was measured as the sum of responses to items (7) "I can always control things that occur to me" and (8) "I have nothing to be proud of" (reverse coded). Openness was measured as the sum of responses to items (9) "Even if I dislike my work, I still do my best to finish it" and (10) "Even if a task takes a long time to achieve the outcome, I still keep up with it."

Control variables were age (interval scale), age-squared, gender, education (with/without college degree), employment status (employed/unemployed), marital status (including married, divorced, separated, widowed, and never married), health status (healthy/unhealthy), residency type (urban and rural) and religion (with or without).

Statistic Model

Because dependent variables and independent variables have various number of missing values, for nested model testing it is crucial to compare model fit with the same sample size. This study adopts list-wise deletion method, the original number of observation is 2,026, the censored observation is 715, and the uncensored observation is 1,311 (final sample size). Since both dependent variables are measured using ordinal scales, and it is crucial to take into account whether list-wise deletion method generates sample selection bias, this study uses the Heckman's ordered probit sample selection model to investigate the relative effects of SES and personality traits on subjective well-being in Taiwan.

Specifically, when analyzing life satisfaction (or happiness), there are two dependent variables in the Heckman's ordered probit sample selection model, one is an ordinal outcome of life satisfaction (or happiness), the other is a binary outcome that indicates whether each observation in the original sample of 2,026 is censored or uncensored in the final sample of 1,311. In the Heckman's ordered probit sample selection model these two dependent variables are jointly determined. This study uses sex, age, marital status and health status as the covariates of selection into the final sample since these four variables have no missing values in the original sample. Simultaneously, the Heckman's model estimates life satisfaction's (or happiness) covariates including different forms of SES, personality traits and the control variables, the results are presented in Tables 6.3 and 6.4 for life satisfaction and happiness, respectively.

Research Findings

Descriptive Statistics

As shown in Table 6.2, for the first dependent variable, the respondents in our sample reported general satisfaction with their lives (mean life satisfaction score of 3.18, maximum = 4.0), about one half of the respondents reported that they are satisfied with their lives (52.94 %), followed by those reported that they are slightly satisfied (22.20 %), that they are slightly unsatisfied (15.03 %), and that they are unsatisfied (9.84 %). For the second dependent variable, the respondents reported general happiness (mean score 1.95, maximum = 3.0), over one half of the respondents reported that they are happy with their life (61.40 %), followed by those who reported that they are unhappy (21.89 %), and that they are very happy (16.70 %).

For the explanatory variables, average self-reported monthly personal income was NT$36,700 (approximately US$ 1,200) and average absolute family income was NT$ 82,300 (approximately US$ 2,800). The majority of respondents felt that their personal incomes were less than they deserve (mean = 2.54) and that their family incomes were insufficient for their necessary expenditures (mean = 2.59). If we look at the objective class structure in Taiwan, approximately half of the Taiwanese are located in the lower non-manual class (48.74 %), the second largest class is lower manual class (18.08 %), followed by upper non-manual class (15.33 %), upper manual class (12.20 %) and farm-related class (5.64 %). On the other hand, when we look at the subjective class structure in Taiwan, 38.60 %

Table 6.2 Sample descriptive statistics

Variable	Mean	SD	Obs	%
Dependent variables				
Life satisfaction	3.18	1.02	1,311	–
Unsatisfied			129	9.84
Slightly unsatisfied			197	15.03
Slightly satisfied			291	22.20
Satisfied			694	52.94
Happiness	1.95	0.62	1,311	–
Unhappy			287	21.89
Happy			805	61.40
Very happy			219	16.70
Explanatory variables				
Absolute income				
Absolute personal income	3.67	3.28	1,311	–
Absolute family income	8.23	7.93	1,311	–
Relative income				
Relative personal income	2.54	0.79	1,311	–
Relative family income	2.59	0.75	1,311	–
Objective class				
Upper non-manual	–	–	201	15.33
Lower non-manual	–	–	639	48.74
Upper manual	–	–	160	12.20
Lower manual	–	–	237	18.08
Farm related	–	–	74	5.64
Subjective class				
Lower class	–	–	91	6.94
Working class	–	–	506	38.60
Lower middle class	–	–	248	18.92
Middle class	–	–	369	28.15
Upper middle class	–	–	97	7.40
Personality				
Extraversion	5.62	0.93	1,311	–
Agreeableness	5.61	0.84	1,311	–
Conscientiousness	6.05	0.93	1,311	–
Emotional stability	5.17	0.83	1,311	–
Openness	6.08	0.92	1,311	–
Control variables				
Age	44.05	14.23	1,311	–
Sex				
Men	–	–	745	56.83
Women	–	–	566	43.17
Education				
High-school and below	–	–	739	56.37
College and above	–	–	572	43.63

(continued)

Table 6.2 (continued)

Variable	Mean	SD	Obs	%
Working status				
Not working	–	–	151	11.52
Working	–	–	1,160	88.48
Marital status				
Never married	–	–	367	27.99
Divorce-separated-widowed	–	–	106	8.09
Married	–	–	838	63.92
Health status				
Healthy	–	–	1,044	79.63
Not healthy	–	–	267	20.37
Residence				
Urban	–	–	689	52.56
Rural	–	–	622	47.44
Religion				
Non	–	–	325	24.79
Yes	–	–	986	75.21

Taiwanese identified themselves as working class, which is the largest share in the class structure, followed by middle class (28.15 %), lower middle class (18.92 %), upper middle class (7.40 %), and lower class (6.94 %). Among the five types of personality trait, the mean score of Openness trait is the highest (mean = 6.08), followed by Conscientiousness trait (6.05), Extraversion trait (5.62), Agreeableness trait (5.61) and Emotional Stability trait (5.17).

Regarding the control variables, the average respondent age was 44.05; 56.83 % of the sample was male and 43.17 % female. Just under half (43.63 %) had university degrees or higher, 88.48 % were employed at the time the survey was conducted, were married (63.92 %), in good health (79.63 %), and practiced a religion (75.21 %). Just over one-half described themselves as urban dwellers (52.56 %).

Ordered Probit Analysis of Life Satisfaction with Sample Selection

Results for the ordered probit analysis of life satisfaction and happiness in Taiwan are shown in Tables 6.3 and 6.4, respectively. All of the models included control variables of age, age-squared, gender, education, work status, marital status, health status, residence, and religion. Model 1 estimates the effect of absolute personal income and family income on life satisfaction (Table 6.3) and happiness (Table 6.4). Model 2 is based on Model 1 but adds the effect of relative personal income and

Table 6.3 Ordered probit regression analysis of life satisfaction

Life satisfaction model	Model 1	Model 2	Model 3	Model 4	Model 5
Explanatory variables					
Absolute personal income	0.034**	0.009	−0.0003	−0.010	−0.012
	(0.012)	(0.014)	(0.014)	(0.015)	(0.015)
Absolute family income	0.014**	0.006	0.006	0.005	0.005
	(0.005)	(0.006)	(0.006)	(0.006)	(0.006)
Relative personal income		0.202***	0.210***	0.220***	0.221***
		(0.039)	(0.040)	(0.040)	(0.040)
Relative family income		0.466***	0.464***	0.448***	0.448***
		(0.045)	(0.046)	(0.045)	(0.045)
Objective class (upper non-manual)					
Lower non-manual			−0.106	−0.051	−0.050
			(0.107)	(0.109)	(0.109)
Upper manual			−0.301*	−0.214	−0.215
			(0.144)	(0.147)	(0.149)
Lower manual			−0.282*	−0.169	−0.165
			(0.134)	(0.136)	(0.138)
Farm-related			−0.469*	−0.305	−0.306
			(0.185)	(0.188)	(0.189)
Subjective class (lower class)					
Working class				0.430**	0.448***
				(0.136)	(0.137)
Lower middle class				0.576***	0.576***
				(0.153)	(0.153)
Middle class				0.660***	0.671***
				(0.153)	(0.154)
Upper middle class				0.917***	0.916***
				(0.201)	(0.203)
Personality					
Extraversion					−0.041
					(0.039)
Agreeableness					0.001
					(0.041)
Conscientiousness					−0.045
					(0.040)
Emotional stability					0.085*
					(0.043)
Openness					0.035
					(0.041)

(continued)

Table 6.3 (continued)

Life satisfaction model	Model 1	Model 2	Model 3	Model 4	Model 5
Control variables					
Age	−0.022	−0.035*	−0.039*	−0.045**	−0.045*
	(0.012)	(0.017)	(0.017)	(0.018)	(0.018)
Age-squared	0.0004**	0.0004**	0.0005**	0.0006***	0.0006***
	(0.0001)	(0.0002)	(0.0002)	(0.0002)	(0.0002)
Sex (men)					
Women	0.473***	0.400***	0.347***	0.324***	0.326***
	(0.060)	(0.096)	(0.101)	(0.097)	(0.099)
Education (high school)					
College and above	0.215***	0.120	0.040	−0.032	−0.038
	(0.066)	(0.080)	(0.086)	(0.089)	(0.089)
Working status (not-W)					
Working	−0.254*	−0.117	−0.036	0.009	0.027
	(0.114)	(0.149)	(0.153)	(0.154)	(0.155)
Marital status (never-M)					
Divorced-S-W	−0.290*	−0.005	0.007	0.046	0.045
	(0.126)	(0.179)	(0.181)	(0.177)	(0.180)
Married	−0.157	0.188	0.191	0.167	0.168
	(0.085)	(0.188)	(0.192)	(0.180)	(0.184)
Health status (healthy)					
Not healthy	−0.498***	−0.524***	−0.522***	−0.517***	−0.517***
	(0.075)	(0.091)	(0.093)	(0.092)	(0.092)
Residence (urban)					
Rural	0.095	0.147*	0.196**	0.243***	0.241***
	(0.052)	(0.068)	(0.071)	(0.072)	(0.072)
Religion (non)					
Yes	0.043	0.082	0.089	0.074	0.073
	(0.062)	(0.078)	(0.078)	(0.079)	(0.079)
Selection model					
Sex (men)					
Women	−0.395***	−0.385***	−0.385***	−0.385***	−0.385***
	(0.058)	(0.059)	(0.059)	(0.059)	(0.059)
Age	−0.017***	−0.018***	−0.018***	−0.018***	−0.018***
	(0.002)	(0.002)	(0.002)	(0.002)	(0.002)
Marital status (never-M)					
Divorced-S-W	0.463***	0.444***	0.444***	0.444***	0.443***
	(0.126)	(0.128)	(0.128)	(0.128)	(0.128)
Married	0.665***	0.681***	0.681***	0.681***	0.681***
	(0.084)	(0.084)	(0.084)	(0.084)	(0.084)

(continued)

Table 6.3 (continued)

Selection model	Model 1	Model 2	Model 3	Model 4	Model 5
Health status (healthy)					
Not healthy	−0.087	−0.066	−0.066	−0.067	−0.067
	(0.069)	(0.071)	(0.071)	(0.071)	(0.071)
Constant	0.932***	0.954***	0.954***	0.955***	0.954***
	(0.090)	(0.091)	(0.091)	(0.091)	(0.091)
Cut point 1	−1.574***	−1.902***	−2.114***	−1.692***	−1.521**
	(0.248)	(0.362)	(0.385)	(0.406)	(0.570)
Cut point 2	−0.997***	−1.139**	1.348***	−0.918*	−0.741
	(0.245)	(0.365)	(0.386)	(0.410)	(0.573)
Cut point 3	−0.466	−0.404	−0.609	−0.170	0.010
	(0.242)	(0.373)	(0.393)	(0.418)	(0.580)
Athrho	−1.628**	−0.234	−0.249	−0.269	−0.253
	(0.547)	(0.450)	(0.462)	(0.428)	(0.437)
Rho	−0.926	−0.230	−0.244	−0.263	−0.248
	(0.078)	(0.426)	(0.435)	(0.398)	(0.410)
Log likelihood	−2,704.08	−2,603.26	−2,598.35	−2,584.92	−2,581.94
Wald chi-square	172.12***	341.32***	344.40***	352.59***	359.92***
LR test of rho = 0, chi-square	5.30*	0.17	0.17	0.21	0.18

*$p < 0.05$, **$p < 0.01$, ***$p < 0.001$
Note: Number of observation = 2,026, censored observation = 715, uncensored observation = 1,311. The statistics in Table 6.3 are coefficient estimates, the statistics in the parentheses are standard errors for the coefficient estimates

family income. Model 3 is based on Model 2 but adds the effect of objective class. Model 4 is based on Model 3 but adds the effect of subjective class. Model 5 is based on Model 4 but adds the effect of personality. Through a series of nested model testing from Model 1 to Model 5 in Tables 6.3 and 6.4, this study tests the relative importance of absolute income, relative income, objective class, subjective class, and personality in explaining life satisfaction and happiness.

Results for Model 1 (the baseline model) indicate that both absolute personal income ($\beta = 0.034$, $p < 0.01$) and absolute family income ($\beta = 0.014$, $p < 0.01$) exerted a highly significant and positive effect on life satisfaction. Model 2 results indicate that the coefficients of relative personal income ($\beta = 0.202$) and relative family income ($\beta = 0.466$) were positive and highly significant ($p < 0.001$). Both absolute income variables were non-significant after relative personal and relative family incomes were added to model 2. Model 3 consisted of comparisons between all of the objective class variables with "upper non-manual class"; the one exception was lower non-manual class. The data indicate that the respondents who described themselves as being in the other three classes felt significantly less life satisfaction. Of the three classes, respondents in the agricultural class had the lowest

Table 6.4 Ordered probit regression analysis of happiness

Happiness model	Model 1	Model 2	Model 3	Model 4	Model 5
Explanatory variables					
Absolute personal income	0.019	−0.002	−0.012	−0.019	−0.025
	(0.013)	(0.013)	(0.014)	(0.014)	(0.014)
Absolute family income	0.0083	0.0005	0.0002	−0.000	0.000
	(0.0051)	(0.0051)	(0.0051)	(0.005)	(0.005)
Relative personal income		0.152***	0.163***	0.168***	0.170***
		(0.038)	(0.039)	(0.039)	(0.039)
Relative family income		0.379***	0.378***	0.365***	0.368***
		(0.039)	(0.040)	(0.041)	(0.041)
Objective class (upper non-manual)					
Lower non-manual			−0.215*	−0.159	−0.150
			(0.101)	(0.103)	(0.103)
Upper manual			−0.356*	−0.273	−0.261
			(0.141)	(0.145)	(0.146)
Lower manual			−0.324*	−0.230	−0.191
			(0.130)	(0.134)	(0.135)
Farm-related			−0.365*	−0.236	−0.211
			(0.182)	(0.186)	(0.188)
Subjective class (lower class)					
Working class				0.221	0.244
				(0.142)	(0.143)
Lower middle class				0.294	0.289
				(0.155)	(0.156)
Middle class				0.383*	0.380*
				(0.155)	(0.156)
Upper middle class				0.676***	0.636**
				(0.192)	(0.194)
Personality					
Extraversion					−0.072
					(0.039)
Agreeableness					0.091*
					(0.041)
Conscientiousness					−0.020
					(0.040)
Emotional stability					0.122**
					(0.043)
Openness					0.032
					(0.041)

(continued)

Table 6.4 (continued)

Happiness model	Model 1	Model 2	Model 3	Model 4	Model 5
Control variables					
Age	−0.027	−0.032	−0.034	−0.037*	−0.036*
	(0.017)	(0.017)	(0.017)	(0.017)	(0.018)
Age-squared	0.0003*	0.0003	0.0003*	0.0004*	0.0004*
	(0.0002)	(0.0002)	(0.0002)	(0.0002)	(0.0002)
Sex (men)					
Women	0.431***	0.363**	0.327*	0.310*	0.318*
	(0.099)	(0.132)	(0.138)	(0.141)	(0.145)
Education (high school)					
College and above	0.248***	0.108	0.030	−0.016	−0.019
	(0.078)	(0.079)	(0.085)	(0.087)	(0.087)
Working status (not-W)					
Working	−.321**	−0.191	−0.128	−0.098	−0.069
	(0.135)	(0.139)	(0.144)	(0.144)	(0.145)
Marital status (never-M)					
Divorced-S-W	−0.127	0.065	0.075	0.099	0.095
	(0.187)	(0.203)	(0.209)	(0.213)	(0.217)
Married	−0.045	0.096	0.093	0.080	0.064
	(0.213)	(0.235)	(0.245)	(0.251)	(0.258)
Health status (healthy)					
Not healthy	−0.428***	−0.314***	−0.314***	−0.312***	−0.302***
	(0.100)	(0.088)	(0.089)	(0.090)	(0.091)
Residence (urban)					
Rural	0.099	0.134*	0.164*	0.190**	0.185**
	(0.065)	(0.067)	(0.070)	(0.070)	(0.071)
Religion (non)					
Yes	0.004	0.022	0.023	0.015	0.017
	(0.076)	(0.079)	(0.079)	(0.079)	(0.080)
Selection model					
Sex (men)					
Women	−0.386***	−0.383***	−0.384***	−0.384***	−0.384***
	(0.060)	(0.059)	(0.059)	(0.059)	(0.059)
Age	−0.018***	−0.018***	−0.018***	−0.018***	−0.018***
	(0.002)	(0.002)	(0.002)	(0.002)	(0.002)
Marital status (never-M)					
Divorced-S-W	0.445***	0.440***	0.440***	0.440***	0.440***
	(0.129)	(0.128)	(0.128)	(0.128)	(0.128)
Married	0.681***	0.680***	0.680***	0.680***	0.680***
	(0.084)	(0.084)	(0.084)	(0.084)	(0.084)

(continued)

Table 6.4 (continued)

Selection model	Model 1	Model 2	Model 3	Model 4	Model 5
Health status (healthy)					
Not healthy	−0.065	−0.064	−0.064	−0.064	−0.064
	(0.070)	(0.071)	(0.071)	(0.071)	(0.071)
Constant	0.952***	0.954***	0.954***	0.953***	0.953***
	(0.091)	(0.091)	(0.091)	(0.091)	(0.091)
Cut point 1	−1.379***	−1.476***	−1.769***	−1.530***	−0.671
	(0.333)	(0.378)	(0.393)	(0.414)	(0.570)
Cut point 2	0.405	0.478	0.192	0.445	1.323*
	(0.383)	(0.394)	(0.412)	(0.439)	(0.594)
Athrho	−0.325	−0.065	−0.084	−0.096	−0.092
	(0.564)	(0.589)	(0.619)	(0.638)	(0.661)
Rho	−0.314	−0.065	−0.083	−0.096	−0.091
	(0.509)	(0.587)	(0.614)	(0.632)	(0.656)
Log likelihood	−2,420.92	−2,354.99	−2,350.81	−2,343.54	−2,334.47
Wald chi-square	109.83***	222.01***	230.46***	243.69***	257.83***
LR test of rho = 0, chi-square	0.14	0.01	0.01	0.01	0.01

*$p < 0.05$, **$p < 0.01$, ***$p < 0.001$

Note: Number of observation = 2,026, censored observation = 715, uncensored observation = 1,311. The statistics in Table 6.4 are coefficient estimates, the statistics in the parentheses are standard errors for the coefficient estimates

life satisfaction (β = −0.469), followed by upper manual (β = −0.301), and lower manual (β = −0.282). Model 3 data also indicated a manual-versus-non-manual division in life satisfaction, with non-manual respondents reporting higher levels of life satisfaction. Model 3 results also indicate a robust effect of relative personal and relative family incomes, with both coefficients highly significant and with virtually identical magnitudes.

Results for Model 4 indicate that all of the subjective class coefficients were highly significant, and that the effect of relative personal and relative family incomes were virtually the same as that noted in Model 3; however, all of the objective class coefficients in Model 4 were non-significant. The subjective class position coefficients indicate a significant class gradient in terms of life satisfaction—that is, the higher the perceived class position, the higher the life satisfaction score, with a large gap between middle class (β = 0.660) and upper middle class respondents (β = 0.917). Regarding Model 5, contrary to our expectations, only emotional stability has a significant and positive effect on life satisfaction (β = 0.085, $p < 0.05$), yet the effects of the relative income and subjective class variables on life satisfaction remained robust throughout.

Regarding the effects of the control variables, the Model 5 results indicate a significant U-shaped age pattern for life satisfaction—that is, we found a negative association between life satisfaction and age (β = −0.045), but to a certain age it actually increased (β = 0.0006). This finding is consistent with those of previous studies (Table 6.3) (for a detailed review of this relationship in the economics literature, see Frey and Stutzer 2002). Women ($\beta = 0.326$) in the sample had an overall higher level of life satisfaction than men, and those living in rural areas ($\beta = 0.241$) reported greater satisfaction with their lives; those who described themselves as unhealthy reported less life satisfaction ($\beta = -0.517$). Respondents with college degrees, who described themselves as religious, and who were married or employed at the time of the survey did not report greater life satisfaction compared to their counterparts at a statistically significant level.

As shown in Table 6.3, the data for Model 1 indicates strong support for H1 since both absolute personal income and absolute family income exert a significant and positive effect on life satisfaction. The Model 2 data of Table 6.3 indicates that relative personal income and relative family income have significant positive effects on life satisfaction net of the effect of absolute personal income and absolute family income; in fact the effect of both types of absolute income disappeared once both types of relative income were included in Model 2. Compared with Model 1, Model 2 has a much better fit since the likelihood-ratio test is highly significant ($\chi^2 = 201.65$, $p = 0.0000$). Accordingly, both H2A and H2B find strong support from the Model 2 results. Next, since the Model 3 data indicate that a majority of objective class variables exerted a positive effect on life satisfaction among the respondents, and compared with Model 2, Model 3 has a better fit since the likelihood-ratio test is significant ($\chi^2 = 9.82$, $p = 0.0435$), H3 is also supported.

Further, despite the positive effect of objective class position on life satisfaction, that effect was substantially diluted when subjective class position was included in Model 4, and compared with Model 3, Model 4 has a better fit since the likelihood-ratio test is significant ($\chi^2 = 26.86$, $p = 0.0000$). This finding suggests that subjective class position plays a highly significant role in determining life satisfaction, and indicates strong support for H4A and H4B. The Model 5 data provide partial support for H5, since only one of the five personality traits (emotional stability) exerted a significant and positive effect on life satisfaction after controlling for the effects of absolute/relative income or objective/subjective class position. Compared with Model 4, Model 5 does not has a better fit since the likelihood-ratio test is not significant ($\chi^2 = 5.97$, $p = 0.3092$), this finding indicates that personality does not have a significant marginal contribution in explaining life satisfaction in Taiwan net of the effect of SES variables.

Table 6.3 includes two parts of the analysis, one is the ordered probit model for the observations which were uncensored in the final sample (without any missing values for all study variables), the other is the selection probit model which determines whether the observations are selected into the final sample. The selection model of Table 6.3 indicates that the likelihood-ratio test statistics for $\rho = 0$ from Model 2 to Model 5 are not significant (except for Model 1), which indicates that the errors for life satisfaction and selection are uncorrelated, and there is no sample selection bias in the analysis of life satisfaction for Taiwanese.

Ordered Probit Analysis of Happiness with Sample Selection

Results for the ordered probit analysis of happiness in Taiwan are presented in Table 6.4. Those for Model 1, the baseline model, indicate non-significance for both the absolute personal and absolute family income variables. However, the Model 2 data indicate that when relative personal income ($\beta = 0.152$) and relative family income ($\beta = 0.379$) were included, both variables became highly significant ($p < 0.001$). In contrast, both absolute income variables were non-significant in Model 2. In Model 3 the coefficients for all objective class variables were significant ($p < 0.05$). Agricultural-related class ($\beta = -0.365$) respondents reported the lowest level of happiness, followed by upper manual ($\beta = -0.356$), lower manual ($\beta = -0.324$), and lower non-manual class ($\beta = -0.215$). Similar to the life satisfaction data shown in Table 6.3, Model 3 also spotlighted a manual-versus-non-manual class divide, with non-manual class respondents reporting higher levels of happiness compared to those in the other social classes. The Model 3 results also reveal robust effects for relative personal and relative family income, with both coefficients highly significant and with essentially equal magnitudes.

In Model 4, the coefficients of two subjective classes were found to be significant. Specifically, respondents identified themselves as middle class or upper middle class reported higher level of happiness than those in the lower class. The effects of relative personal and relative family income were virtually identical to those in Model 3, while all of the objective class coefficients were non-significant. Similar to life satisfaction analytical results, the subjective class coefficient in Model 4 indicated a significant and clearly identifiable class gradient for happiness: the higher the perceived class position, the greater the degree of happiness, with a large gap between self-described middle class ($\beta = 0.383$) and upper middle class respondents ($\beta = 0.676$). For Model 5, the coefficients of two types of personality traits were significant: respondents with high scores in agreeableness ($\beta = 0.091$) and emotional stability ($\beta = 0.122$) reported higher levels of happiness. The Model 5 results also confirmed robust effects of the relative income and subjective class variables on happiness.

Regarding the effects of the control variables (Table 6.4), Model 5 displayed a significantly U-shaped age pattern indicating a negative relationship between age and happiness ($\beta = -0.036$); however, up to a certain age, happiness increased with age ($\beta = 0.0004$), which is consistent with previous reports as reviewed by Frey and Stutzer (2002). The same results also indicate that the female respondents ($\beta = 0.318$) tended to report greater happiness than the males, that respondents living in rural areas ($\beta = 0.185$) reported greater happiness than those living in urban areas, and healthy respondents reporting greater happiness than their unhealthy counterparts ($\beta = -0.302$). However, no significant differences were found for marriage, college degree, working status, or religious affiliation.

Looking at Table 6.4, the Model 1 results indicate no significant effects for absolute personal or absolute family income, confirming that H1 is not supported by the data. The Model 2 results indicate significant and positive effects for both relative personal and relative family income on happiness net of the effect of absolute personal and absolute family income. Compared with Model 1, Model 2 has a much better fit since the likelihood-ratio test is highly significant ($\chi^2 = 131.87$, $p = 0.0000$), and as in Model 1, the effects of both types of absolute income were non-significant, thus giving strong support to H2A and H2B. The Model 3 data show that all objective class variables exerted a positive effect on happiness among the respondents, thus supporting H3. Compared with Model 2, Model 3 does not has a better fit since the likelihood-ratio test is not significant ($\chi^2 = 8.37$, $p = 0.0790$), this finding indicates that net of the effect of absolute and relative income variables, the inclusion of objective class variables in Model 3 does not have substantial marginal contribution in explaining the happiness of Taiwanese.

Even though objective class position exerted a positive effect on happiness, when subjective class position was included in Model 4, the effect of objective class position completely disappeared, while subjective class position continued to play a role in determining happiness; since only two subjective class variables are significant, these findings give partial support to H4A and H4B. Compared with Model 3, Model 4 has a better fit since the likelihood-ratio test is significant ($\chi^2 = 14.54$, $p = 0.0058$), this finding indicates that net of the effect of absolute and relative income variables, and objective class variables, the inclusion of subjective class variables have significant marginal contribution in explaining the happiness of Taiwanese. Finally, H5 is partially supported by the Model 5 data shown in Table 6.4, since agreeableness and emotional stability were found to exert a significant positive effect on happiness of the respondents controlling for the effects of absolute/relative income and objective/subjective class position. Compared with Model 4, Model 5 has a better fit since the likelihood-ratio test is significant ($\chi^2 = 18.13$, $p = 0.0028$), this finding indicates that personality has a significant marginal contribution in explaining the happiness of Taiwanese net of the effect of SES variables.

As in Table 6.3, Table 6.4 also includes two parts of the analysis, one is the ordered probit model for the observations which were uncensored in the analysis of happiness, the other is the selection probit model which determines whether the observations are selected into the final sample. The selection model of Table 6.4 indicates that the likelihood-ratio test statistics for $\rho = 0$ from Model 1 to Model 5 are not significant, which indicates that the errors for happiness and selection are uncorrelated, and there is no sample selection bias in the analysis of happiness for Taiwanese.

Discussion

The results of this study imply that the way people evaluate where they stand in regard to the income and class position along the SES ladder matters more than the actual standing in terms of absolute income and objective class in determining subjective well-being. Our analysis renders little support for the *Absolute Theory*, since absolute income does not have any significant effect net of relative income. For the effect of relative income, the results are consistent with the prediction of the *Aspiration Theory*, that is, regardless of the level of absolute income, the degree of individual well-being is strongly affected by individual's expectation that people think how well they deserved in terms of relative income. The results are also consistent with the prediction of the *Relative Theory*, that is, regardless the level of absolute income and objective class position, individual well-being is strongly affected by the relative success an individual perceived in terms of income and class position along the social ladders.

On the other hand, this study provides only moderate support for the *Adaptation Theory*, since personality trait in our analysis only has partial effects on life satisfaction and happiness. In a nutshell, the analysis of this study suggests a very strong influence of socio-psychological dimensions of socioeconomic status (e.g. relative income and subjective class) in determining individual well-being; and subjective explanatory variables are more important than objective explanatory variables in predicting individual well-being, which is also a subjective dependent variable. The analysis of this study is consistent with previous studies (Cummins 2000).

Conclusions and Future Research Direction

The findings of the final model in this study (based on Model 5) show that the effects of social demographic characteristics are important determinants of subjective well-being in Taiwan. Specifically, results for Model 5 in the analysis of life satisfaction and happiness indicate a significant U-shaped age pattern on subjective well-being. Moreover, women in the sample and those living in rural areas reported higher level of SWB, whereas unhealthy respondents reported lower level of SWB. These findings are consistent with previous study by Okulicz-Kozaryn (2011), who used GSS data and found women are happier than men, and married or healthy respondents report higher level of happiness, and a significant U-shaped age pattern of happiness in the U.S. These results highlight the importance of social demographic characteristics as control variables in the analysis of subjective well-being.

Regarding explanatory variables, income does matter when it comes to subjective well-being in terms of life satisfaction and happiness in Taiwan. The results for Model 2 in Tables 6.3 and 6.4 indicate that, after taking into account the effect of relative income, absolute personal income and family income have no significant effects on life satisfaction and happiness, whereas relative personal and family incomes become highly significant.

In addition to taking into account of income, the class dimension of SES characteristics is also crucial. For class effects, the analysis for Model 3 shows that objective class position has significant and strong effects on life satisfaction and happiness, and there is manual versus non-manual class divide in life satisfaction and happiness. However, the analysis of life satisfaction and happiness for Model 4 indicates that, once subjective class position is taking into account, the effect of objective class position was virtually diluted by the effect of subjective class position. Similar to the effect of objective class position, the effect of subjective class position indicates a significant and clear class gradient of life satisfaction and happiness, that is, the higher the perceived class position toward the top of the class structure, the higher the degree of subjective well-being.

The results for Model 5 in Tables 6.3 and 6.4 reveals that socioeconomic status in terms of income and class has much stronger effects than that of personality trait on subjective well-being in Taiwan. Specifically, the Model 5 of this study found after taking into account the effect of SES (income and class) and socio-demographic characteristics only one personality trait (Emotional Stability) has a significant positive effect on life satisfaction, and two personality traits (Agreeableness and Emotional Stability) have a significant positive effect on happiness in Taiwan. Our results are consistent with studies using large and representative surveys (Helliwell 2006), which often found very moderate effect of personality traits on subjective well-being, after taking into account relevant covariates such as trust and religiosity.

On a whole, this study found that there are significant SES (income and class) gradients of subjective well-being, whereas personality traits play moderate role in determining subjective well-being. Future research agenda needs to explore the following issues. First, although we found net of relative income, there are no significant effects of absolute income on well-being (as in Model 2) and the fact that the effect of objective class position become disappear once the analysis includes subjective class position (as in Model 4), does this really mean that absolute income or objective class position has no effect on subjective well-being? It might be possible that there are more complex mechanisms that have translated objective explanatory variables (such as absolute income or objective class) into some important subjective variables, such as self-rated health status, which directly affect individual well-being. For example, Oishi et al. (2011) using GSS survey data from 1972 to 2008 to examine the relationship between income inequality and happiness in the U.S., they found that Americans were on average happier in years with less income inequality for lower-income respondents, but not for higher-income respondents. The negative association between income inequality and happiness among lower-income Americans was mainly explained by their perceived unfairness and lack of trust, instead of lower family income. Future research needs more analyses to explore the possibilities of such causal mechanisms (the indirect effect of absolute income and objective class position) on subjective well-being in Taiwan.

Second, this study found absolute incomes do not have significant effects on subjective well-being in Taiwan after taking into account the effect of relative incomes, it may be that absolute incomes and individual well-being have a nonlinear, instead of linear, relationship. According to Veenhoven's *Absolute Theory* (1988), below the threshold income level, an increase of absolute income shall increase individual well-being since human basic needs have been satisfied by income; however, beyond the threshold income, the positive effect of income on well-being tends to diminish and level off since individual's marginal utility is decreasing when human basic needs are no longer a problem. Future research could further investigate the threshold effect of absolute income on well-being in Taiwan.

Third, one major findings of this study is that socioeconomic status is more important than personality traits in explaining subjective well-being in Taiwan; however, as Lucas (2008) and Albuquerque et al. (2012) pointed out the ambiguous status of the causal link between personality traits and subjective well-being, future studies need to engage more detailed analysis of the mechanism involved in the causal link, including the collection of more refined measures of personality trait in large representative survey sample that allow more detailed analysis of the effect of personality trait on well-being. Moreover, future research could benefit from the investigation of more refined measures of relative socioeconomic status (such as income and class) that takes into account the process of social comparison. For example, what is the reference group an individual compare with when evaluating their relative success? Recent studies have made a good case in explaining the differential effect of neighborhood on subjective well-being when making social comparison (Firebaugh and Schroeder 2009; Hou 2014).

Acknowledgements This study was supported by a project entitled 'Temporal and Cross-National Analysis of Quality of Life: The Effects of Socioeconomic Status, Working Conditions, Personal Characteristics, and Social Relations.' From the National Science Council to Hsiu-Jen Yeh (NSC 101-2410-H-194-070). Additional support came from a Tunghai University GREEnS project entitled 'Enhancing the Quality of Life and Living Environment in an Ageing Society.' Many thanks to the reviewers for their constructive suggestions. We thank Li-Hsueh Wu and Tzu-Chuan Tsai for their excellent work of data computing.

References

Academia Sinica. (2014). *Taiwan Social Change Survey*. http://www.ios.sinica.edu.tw/sc/en/home2.php. Accessed 5 June 2014.

Akerlof, G. (1997). Social distance and social decisions. *Econometrica, 65*, 1005–1027.

Akerlof, G., & Kranton, R. (2000). Economics and identity. *Quarterly Journal of Economics, 115*, 715–753.

Akerlof, G., & Kranton, R. (2010). *Identity economics*. Princeton: Princeton University Press.

Albuquerque, I., Pedroso de Lima, M., Matos, M., & Figueiredo, C. (2012). Personality and subjective well-being: What hides behind global analyses? *Social Indicators Research, 105*, 447–460.

Argyle, M. (1999). Causes and correlates of happiness. In D. Kahneman, E. Diener, & N. Schwarz (Eds.), *Well-being: The foundations of hedonic psychology* (pp. 213–229). New York: Russell Sage.

Brennan, G. (1973). Pareto desirable redistribution: The case of malice and envy. *Journal of Public Economics, 2*, 173–183.

Brickman, P., & Campbell, D. T. (1971). Hedonic relativism and planning the good society. In M. H. Appley (Ed.), *Adaptation-level theory: A symposium* (pp. 287–302). New York: Academic.

Brickman, P., Coates, D., & Janoff-Bulman, R. (1978). Lottery winners and accident victims: Is happiness relative? *Journal of Personality and Social Psychology, 36*, 917–927.

Chang, L. Y. (2011). Are they happy? And why? Taiwan and Hong Kong in comparison, 2000~2005. In M. H. H. Hsiao, P. S. Wan, & T. K. Y. Wong (Eds.), *Interpreting the social ethos of Taiwan and Hong Kong* (pp. 33–55). Hong Kong: Hong Kong Institute of Asia-Pacific Studies.

Chang, W. C. (2013). Climbing up the social ladders: Identity, relative income, and subjective well-being. *Social Indicators Research, 113*(1), 513–535.

Clark, A. E., Frijters, P., & Shields, M. A. (2008). Relative income, happiness, and utility: An explanation for the Easterlin Paradox and other puzzles. *Journal of Economic Literature, 46*, 95–144.

Costa, P. T., & McCrae, R. R. (1980). Influence of extraversion and neuroticism on subjective well-being: Happy and unhappy people. *Journal of Personality and Social Psychology, 38*, 668–678.

Cummins, R. A. (2000). Personal income and subjective well-being: A review. *Journal of Happiness Studies, 1*, 133–158.

DeNeve, K. M., & Cooper, H. (1998). The happy personality: A meta-analysis of 137 personality traits and subjective well-being. *Psychological Bulletin, 124*, 197–229.

Diener, E., & Diener, C. (1996). Most people are happy. *Journal of Psychological Science, 7*(3), 181–185.

Diener, E., & Lucas, R. E. (1999). Personality and subjective well-being. In D. Kahneman, E. Diener, & N. Schwartz (Eds.), *Well-being: The foundation of hedonic psychology* (pp. 213–229). New York: Russell Sage.

Dolan, P., Peasgood, T., & White, M. (2008). Do we really know what makes us happy? A review of the economic literature on the factors associated with subjective well-being. *Journal of Economic Psychology, 29*, 94–122.

Duesenberry, J. S. (1949). *Income, savings and the theory of consumer behavior*. Cambridge, MA: Harvard University Press.

Durayappah, A. (2011). The 3P model: A general theory of subjective well-being. *Journal of Happiness Studies, 12*(4), 681–716.

Durkheim, E. (1897). *Suicide: A study in sociology*. Glencoe: Free Press.

Easterlin, R. A. (1974). Does economic growth improve the human lot? Some empirical evidence. In M. Abramovitz, P. A. David, & M. W. Reder (Eds.), *Nations and households in economic growth* (pp. 89–125). New York: Academic.

Easterlin, R. A. (1995). Will raising the incomes of all increase the happiness of all? *Journal of Economic Behavior & Organization, 27*, 35–47.

Easterlin, R. A. (2001). Income and happiness: Towards a unified theory. *Economic Journal, 111*, 465–484.

Firebaugh, G., & Schroeder, M. B. (2009). Does your neighbor's income affect your happiness? *American Journal of Sociology, 115*(3), 805–831.

Frank, R. H. (1985). *Choosing the right pond: Human behavior and the quest for status*. New York: Oxford University Press.

Frey, B. S., & Stutzer, A. (2002). *Happiness and economics*. Princeton: Princeton University Press.

Fuentes, N., & Rojas, M. (2001). Economic theory and subjective well-being: Mexico. *Social Indicators Research, 53*(3), 289–314.

Funder, D. C., & Fast, L. A. (2010). Personality in social psychology. In S. T. Fiske, D. T. Gilbert, & G. Lindsey (Eds.), *Handbook of social psychology* (5th ed., pp. 668–697). New York: Wiley.

Gitmez, A. S., & Morcöl, G. (1994). Socio-economic status and life satisfaction in Turkey. *Social Indicators Research, 31*(1), 77–98.

Gosling, S. D., Rentfrow, P. J., & Swann, W. B., Jr. (2003). A very brief measure of the big-five personality domains. *Journal of Research in Personality, 37*, 504–528.

Ha, S. E., & Kim, S. (2013). Personality and subjective well-being: Evidence from South Korea. *Social Indicators Research, 111*, 341–359.

Helliwell, J. F. (2006). Well-being, social capital, and public policy: What's new? *Economic Journal, 116*, C34–C45.

Helson, H. (1964). *Adaptation-level theory*. New York: Harper & Row.

Hou, F. (2014). Keep up with the Joneses or keep on as their neighbours: Life satisfaction and income in Canadian urban neighbourhoods. *Journal of Happiness Studies, 15*(5), 1085–1107. doi:10.1007/s10902-013-9465-4.

House, J. S. (1981). Social structure and personality. In M. Rosenberg & R. Turner (Eds.), *Sociological perspectives on social psychology* (pp. 525–561). New York: Basic Books.
Hout, M., & Greeley, A. M. (2012). Religion and happiness. In P. V. Marsden (Ed.), *Social trends in American life* (pp. 288–314). Princeton: Princeton University Press.
John, O. P., Naumann, L. P., & Soto, C. J. (2008). Paradigm shift to the integrative big five trait taxonomy: History, measurement, and conceptual issues. In O. P. John, R. W. Robins, & L. A. Pervin (Eds.), *Handbook of personality: Theory and research* (3rd ed., pp. 114–158). New York: Guilford.
Liao, P. S., Fu, Y. C., & Yi, C. C. (2005). Perceived quality of life in Taiwan and Hong Kong: An intra-culture comparison. *Journal of Happiness Studies, 6*, 43–67.
Lu, L., Kao, S. F., Chang, T. T., Wu, H. P., & Cooper, C. L. (2011). Work/family demands, work flexibility, work/family conflict, and their consequences at work: A national probability sample in Taiwan. *International Perspectives in Psychology: Research, Practice, Consultation, 1*(S), 68–81.
Lucas, R. E. (2008). Personality and subjective well-being. In M. Eid & R. J. Larsen (Eds.), *The science of subjective well-being* (pp. 171–194). New York: The Guilford Press.
Luttmer, E. (2005). Neighbors as negatives: Relative earnings and well-being. *Quarterly Journal of Economics, 120*, 963–1002.
Lykken, D., & Tellegen, A. (1996). Happiness is a stochastic phenomenon. *Psychological Science, 7*, 186–189.
Meadow, H. L., Metzer, J., Rahtz, D. R., & Sirgy, M. J. (1992). A life satisfaction measure based on judgment theory. *Social Indicators Research, 26*, 23–59.
Mirowsky, J., & Ross, C. E. (1986). Social patterns of distress. *Annual Review of Sociology, 12*(1), 23–45.
NORC. (2014). *General Social Survey*. http://www3.norc.org/gss+website. Accessed 5 June 2014.
Oishi, S., Kesebir, S., & Diener, E. (2011). Income inequality and happiness. *Psychological Science, 22*(9), 1095–1100.
Okulicz-Kozaryn, A. (2011). Europeans work to live and Americans live to work (who is happy to work more: Americans or Europeans?). *Journal of Happiness Studies, 12*, 225–243.
Oswald, A. (1997). Happiness and economic performance. *Economic Journal, 107*, 1815–1831.
Parducci, A. (1982, August). *Toward a relational theory of happiness*. Paper presented at the 90th annual convention of the American Psychological Association, Washington, DC.
Roberts, B. W. (2009). Back to the future: Personality and assessment and personality development. *Journal of Research in Personality, 43*, 137–145.
Schnittker, J. (2008). Happiness and success: Genes, families, and the psychological effects of socioeconomic position and social support. *American Journal of Sociology, 114*(Suppl), S233–S259.
Schooler, C. (1984). Psychological effects of complex environments during the life span: A review and theory. *Intelligence, 8*, 259–281.
Tsai, M. C. (2007). Does globalization affect human well-being? *Social Indicators Research, 81*, 102–126.
Tsai, M. C. (2009). Market openness, transition economies and subjective wellbeing. *Journal of Happiness Studies, 10*, 523–539.
Tsai, M. C., Chang, H. H., & Chen, W. C. (2012). Globally happy: Individual globalization, expanded capacities, and subjective wellbeing. *Social Indicators Research, 108*, 509–524.
Tsou, M. W., & Liu, J. T. (2001). Happiness and domain satisfaction in Taiwan. *Journal of Happiness Studies, 2*(3), 269–288.
Veblen, T. (1899). *The theory of the leisure class*. New York/London: George Allen and Unwin/Macmillan.
Veenhoven, R. (1988). The utility of happiness? *Social Indicators Research, 20*, 334–354.
Veenhoven, R. (2000). The four qualities of life. *Journal of Happiness Studies, 1*, 1–39.
Yang, Y. (2008). Social inequalities in happiness in the United States, 1972 to 2004: An age-period-cohort analysis. *American Sociological Review, 73*(1), 204–226.
Yeh, H. J. (2015). Job demands, job resources, and job satisfaction in East Asia. *Social Indicators Research, 121*, 47–60. doi:10.1007/s11205-014-0631-9.

Chapter 7
The Impact of Government Size on Chinese Elders' Life Satisfaction: 1998–2008

Song Gao and Xiangyi Meng

Introduction

The main purpose of this article is to investigate the impact of government size on individual life satisfaction in China during a period of rapid income growth and wealth accumulation. It has been documented that there has been a declining trend in the average Subjective Well-being (SWB) of Chinese over periods of spectacular economic growth (Brockmann et al. 2009 for 1990–2000 and Easterlin et al. 2012 for 1990–2010).[1] With this observation, a natural question arises: what could be the negative factors in Chinese lives that offset the positive impact (if any) of income growth? Although data is quite limited in Easterlin et al. (2012) study (small sample size, limited geographical coverage and mainly urban), the authors have tried to draw a causal link for this observation: "the inverse change in unemployment, dissolution of the social safety net and growing income inequality have reduced Chinese life satisfaction in spite of massive improvement in average living standards."

Potentially there might be more factors that could negatively influence individuals' life satisfaction. In the literature several candidate factors such as government size and inequality have been empirically tested since Easterlin's seminal work (Easterlin 1974), the main implication from which has been named "Easterlin Paradox", that is, *growth without happiness* (at least after a threshold of per

[1] Other researchers find a "flat line" (for example, Crabtree and Wu (2011)'s Gallup report for 1999–2010).

S. Gao • X. Meng (✉)
China Academy of Public Finance and Policy, The Central University of Finance and Economics, No. 39 Xueyuan Nanlu, Haidian District, Beijing 100081, China
e-mail: song.gao@cufe.edu.cn; song.gao@gmail.com; xiangyi.meng@cufe.edu.cn; danielxymeng@gmail.com

F. Maggino (ed.), *A New Research Agenda for Improvements in Quality of Life*, Social Indicators Research Series 57, DOI 10.1007/978-3-319-15904-1_7

capita GDP).[2] First, there has been a significant empirical literature on individuals' preferences over unemployment, inflation and inequality using happiness/life satisfaction surveys (see Di Tella et al. 2001, 2003; Alesina et al. 2004). This line of research presents econometric evidence that some main macroeconomic variables including unemployment, inflation and inequality all negatively affect individuals' life satisfaction/happiness, even after controlling for a rich set of personal characteristics.

Second, there has been a relatively small but increasing amount of research on the relationship between government activities and individual life satisfaction. The principal idea is that, according to public choice theory, the actual government size might not be lined up with individuals' preferences, due to either information shortcomings or special interest groups or both (Frey and Stutzer 2010). For example, Bjørnskov et al. (2007) find a significantly negative partial correlation between government consumption as a percentage of GDP and life satisfaction using a cross-section sample of 74 countries. Yamamura (2011) also finds that government expenditure as a percentage of GDP detrimentally affects life satisfaction when government size impedes economic growth. In contrast, Di Tella and MacCulloch (2006) find a positive but insignificant impact of government size on life satisfaction in ten European countries. It seems that the hypothesis of a negative impact of government size on life satisfaction remains an empirical question, as public choice theory points to both positive and negative impacts (Frey and Stutzer 2010).

Following the second line of research, the main purpose of this paper is to investigate the impact on Chinese subjective well-being (SWB) of government size. We are going to employ both provincial and time variations to identify the potential impact.

Happiness Research in China

Almost all research on the economics of Chinese happiness has been focused on individual determinants. As is clearly summarized in Knight and Gunatilaka (2011), the main findings are: (1) current income is a significantly positive predictor of happiness; (2) both relative income and aspiration matter, and the impacts are influenced by people's reference groups and reference times; (3) Income expectations are important for current happiness (Liu and Shang 2012 for urban China).

Brockmann et al. (2009), setting out to explain the declining happiness in China over the 1990–2000 decade, find that financial dissatisfaction is a more important

[2] Several theories such as relative position hypothesis and aspiration theory have been raised and subsequently tested by many researchers. (See survey papers by Frey and Stutzer 2002; Di Tella and MacCulloch 2006; Kahneman and Krueger 2006; Clark et al. 2008).

factor in depressing happiness than other negative feelings emerging with rapid transition, such as anomie and political disaffection.

As far as we know, our paper is the first to look at the impact on Chinese SWB of government size. The main reason is possibly due to the lack of time series data. To robustly investigate these potential impacts for Chinese, a nationally representative longitudinal data at the individual (household) level will be ideal. However, such data are very rare and most of them in China are just 1 year cross-section sample (see Knight and Gunatilaka 2011 for a review on a series of studies.)

There are very few data that track Chinese life satisfaction/happiness consistently over time. World Values Survey is an exception but with a small sample size, which varies between 1,000 and 2,000 individuals for 1990, 1995, 2001 and 2007; when we look at government size at the province level, there are only a few dozens of individuals from each province, which can not provide enough precision on these aggregate variables in our econometric analysis and will further stop us from doing any decomposition along finer geographic/demographic classification, say urban versus rural or east versus west. In this paper we are able to use a large repeated cross section survey of elders, which has a large sample size (roughly over 10,000 individuals each year), covers a large geographic area (22 provinces out of 31 in total) and includes both rural and urban residents. Although elders (65 plus) are only a subpopulation of Chinese, the merits of this data set introduced as above outweigh.

On the other hand, population aging is an increasingly important public issue. Recent statistics[3] shows that elders of 60 (65) and above account for 13.7 % (8.87 %) of the total population by the end of 2011 and it has been projected that this percentage of elders will increase to 35 % by 2053. As a result, elders as a subgroup of the society will be of great concern to the economy and fiscal policies that are targeted at ensuring their welfare. Therefore, to understand the relationship between government size and individual SWB in China, this data set is arguably the most suitable one as far as we know.

Data

This study uses survey data from the Chinese Longitudinal Healthy Longevity Survey (CLHLS), conducted in 1998, 2000, 2002, 2005 and 2008, which aims to investigate the determinants of healthy longevity of human beings. The survey re-interviews survivors at each wave and replaces the deceased with new participants to make a longitudinal dataset which covers a variety of questions including demographic, socioeconomic, behavioral, biological, and environmental factors. This survey covers a randomly selected half of all the counties and cities in 22 Chinese provinces, representing 85 % of the total Chinese population, and has conducted approximately 70,000 interviews on the elders (aged 65 plus) and 10,000 on middle-age adults (aged 35–64).[4] We drop the

[3] http://finance.ce.cn/rolling/201210/23/t20121023_16996977.shtml, accessed on March 23, 2015

[4] http://centerforaging.duke.edu/design-and-method/survey-design

middle-age adults because they were interviewed in only 8 provinces. Further by dropping the subsample of those being cognitively impaired, we restrict our analysis to cognitively normal people. Finally our sample includes 6,773 individuals in 1998, 8,210 in 2000, 12,103 in 2002, 11,693 in 2005, and 11,895 in 2008.[5]

The main dependent variable in this study is the life satisfaction that reads "How do you rate your life at present? – very good, good, so so, bad, or very bad?" (the small "not able to answer" category is not studied here). This question was under the session of "life satisfaction and personality" and was asked consistently in all five waves of the survey. Due to the small number of observations of feeling "very bad" (0.61 %) about life, we collapse the bottom two categories (very bad and bad) into one as "bad". Moreover, we recode the "life satisfaction" variable as 1 if feeling bad, 2 if so so, 3 if good and 4 if very good. The explanatory variables include two major groups – macroeconomic variables and individual socio-economic characteristics. To control for the macroeconomic variables, we use GDP per capita (inflation adjusted, in 1,000 *yuan*), the percentage of government consumption out of GDP, the percentage of capital formation out of GDP, and the per capita expenditure on public health (*yuan*) at provincial level in each survey year. The former three variables measure the government's involvement in the economy and the latter variable relates the most interesting aspect to the older population. These data come from the annual statistics released by the National Bureau of Statistics of China (NBS).

The individual socio-economic variables are drawn from the CLHLS including gender (male = 1), age (65–79, 80–90, 90–100, 100+), ethnicity (Han = 1), education achievement (illiterate, primary school, middle school), occupation before retirement (white collar = 1), living arrangement (living alone, only with spouse, only with children, with spouse and children, with others other than spouse and children, in an institution), children paying frequent visits (yes = 1), sibling paying frequent visits (yes = 1), the number of chronic conditions (hypertension, diabetes, heart disease, stroke, asthma, lung disease, or cancer), the number of ADLs (difficulty in bathing, dressing, toileting, indoor transferring, continence, or eating), income quartile (25th = 1, 50th = 2, 75th = 3, 100th = 4), and self-rated economic position (rich, fair, poor). We also include the province and year dummies to control for province-specific time-constant factors and aggregate shocks to all provinces.

We combine the macro-level data with the CLHLS individual data together by each interviewee's residence (province) and interview time (wave). We further split the sample in three different ways. First, we split the sample into urban and rural areas because huge inequality exists between urban and rural China in terms of income, benefits, and welfares. Second, we split the sample into east and central/west areas which are quite different in terms of economic development. Finally, we split the sample into two groups of rich and poor according to their household per capita income.

[5] The cognitive status of interviewees is determined using the mini-mental state examination (MMSE; Folstein et al. 1975). The MMSE score ranges from 0 to 30, and people with scores of 18 or more are considered as being cognitively normal and those with scores less than 18 are categorized as cognitively impaired (Zeng et al. 2002). Cognitively impaired elders are dropped because they may not be able to appropriately address their feelings about life satisfaction.

Table 7.1 Life satisfaction in China: 1998–2008

		Year				
Reported life satisfaction	All	1998	2000	2002	2005	2008
Bad	5.02	2.62	3.83	5.82	5.77	5.65
So so	30.29	21.92	27.00	32.63	32.40	32.83
Good	47.83	55.39	46.55	46.50	46.31	47.31
Very good	16.86	20.07	22.61	15.05	15.52	14.22
	Region		Residence		Economic Status	
Reported life satisfaction	East	West	Urban	Rural	Rich	Poor
Bad	4.48	5.84	3.90	6.02	3.23	7.71
So so	30.44	30.05	28.00	32.33	28.65	35.95
Good	46.27	50.21	47.46	48.17	49.66	44.25
Very good	18.81	13.90	20.65	13.48	18.47	12.08

Based on 50,674 observations. All numbers are expressed as a percentage

Table 7.1 reports some basic statistics for our subsamples by urban/rural residence, regional areas, and income groups. We define the subsample as rich if the household's per capita income in the residential province was above the median level and as poor if below the median. According to the geographical and economical division in China, Beijing, Tianjin, Liaoning, Shanghai, Jiangsu, Zhejiang, Fujian, Shandong and Guangdong provinces are categorized as east area, and the other provinces are considered as central or west areas. Central and west areas have much similarity in terms of macro- and socio-economic characteristics. Therefore we group these provinces together as one group – central/west area.

Table 7.1 shows that the overall life satisfaction of the elder declined during 1998–2008 – a rapid economic development period, especially after 2000. Since 2002, the level of life satisfaction appeared relatively stable. It is interesting to notice that the elders' life satisfaction in the east and central/west areas did not show significant differences except that more eastern elders felt good about their lives while more central/western elders felt very good. In other words, western elders were slightly happier than their eastern counterparts during this period. This regional difference for the elders is significantly different from that of working age adults who demonstrate completely the opposite (Gao et al. 2014). As expected, urban residents were much happier about their lives than their rural counterparts. And not surprisingly, the rich felt more satisfied than the poor.

Table 7.2 summarizes GDP growth and the government involvement in the economy during 1998 and 2008. The overall GDP per capita undoubtedly had an increasing trend over these years and the growth rate remained high. The eastern GDP more than doubles the central/western GDP. The government consumption was only about 13–14 % of GDP and it shows an inverse U shape over 10 years. There is no significant difference between eastern and central/western areas in terms of government consumption. In contrast, the rate of capital formation exhibits a U shape with a decreasing trend in earlier years and an increasing one in later years. Although GDP grew very fast in this period, the government spending on public health did not grow as fast as GDP in the initial few years between 1998 and

Table 7.2 GDP and government involvement in the economy in China: 1998–2008

	Year	Overall	East	Central/West
GDP per capita (1,000 *yuan*)	1998	8.06	11.28	4.98
	2000	8.67	12.27	5.06
	2002	9.02	12.83	5.21
	2005	10.81	15.18	6.44
	2008	12.66	17.30	8.02
Government consumption/GDP (%)	1998	12.18	11.64	12.70
	2000	13.62	13.22	14.03
	2002	14.66	14.58	14.75
	2005	13.56	13.84	13.27
	2008	13.19	13.47	12.91
Capital formation/GDP (%)	1998	43.31	45.37	41.35
	2000	41.65	43.06	40.25
	2002	42.06	42.49	41.63
	2005	47.62	47.35	47.88
	2008	52.59	49.27	55.90
Per capita Government expenditure on public health (*yuan*)	1998	41.54	60.52	23.43
	2000	46.33	66.60	26.05
	2002	46.94	68.10	25.78
	2005	57.02	81.07	32.97
	2008	103.41	131.18	75.64

2002. We observe a large increase in 2005 followed by a dramatic fall in 2008 in both eastern and central/western China.

Table 7.3 provides the summaries of sample statistics which show the change of household demographics over time. We find that more elders lived alone or with spouse only and that their tendency to live with children only weakened significantly over time. This testifies the "Empty Nest" phenomenon of the elders in China. At the same time, there is an increasing trend of frequent visits by children and siblings which both might improve the elders' life satisfaction. Health is another important factor impacting people's life satisfaction. Our sample shows that over this period the average number of chronic conditions increased along with a decrease in the difficulty of activities of daily living.

It is interesting to notice that over time people were less likely to feel rich and more likely to feel poor even though the household per capita income increased significantly during the same period.[6] This might imply a decreasing satisfaction about their relative economic status.

---

[6] The CLHLS started to question about household income and self-rated economic status since 2002. The question reads "What was the income per capita of your household last year?" in 2002 and 2005, then it was rephrased as "What was the total income of your household last year?" in 2008. Therefore we use income quartiles to replace the real household per capita income in the analysis.

Table 7.3 Sample summary statistics: 1998–2008

	All	Year				
		1998	2000	2002	2005	2008
Observations	50,674	6,773	8,210	12,103	11,693	11,895
Male	0.477	0.464	0.466	0.473	0.478	0.493
Age						
65–79	0.269	0.019	0.004	0.391	0.407	0.368
80–89	0.353	0.482	0.530	0.296	0.274	0.295
90–99	0.251	0.323	0.328	0.198	0.223	0.236
100+	0.119	0.176	0.138	0.115	0.096	0.101
Han	0.938	0.929	0.939	0.944	0.944	0.932
Education						
Illiterate	0.562	0.604	0.584	0.557	0.549	0.541
Primary	0.316	0.279	0.308	0.319	0.324	0.331
Middle	0.118	0.112	0.103	0.119	0.124	0.126
White collar	0.096	0.095	0.089	0.104	0.101	0.087
Living arrangement						
Alone	0.141	0.113	0.131	0.139	0.142	0.165
Institution	0.038	0.054	0.071	0.042	0.023	0.016
With spouse only	0.184	0.098	0.115	0.196	0.223	0.231
With children only	0.480	0.609	0.562	0.449	0.446	0.417
With S & C	0.126	0.090	0.091	0.151	0.144	0.126
With others	0.031	0.036	0.029	0.023	0.023	0.046
Child paying frequent visits	0.822	0.725	0.756	0.857	0.833	0.877
Sibling paying frequent visits	0.291	0.183	0.205	0.245	0.312	0.439
# Chronic conditions	0.466	0.394	0.392	0.475	0.510	0.505
# ADLs	0.386	0.583	0.492	0.408	0.321	0.244

(continued)

Table 7.3 (continued)

	All	Year				
		1998	2000	2002	2005	2008
Perceived economic status						
Rich	0.169	–	–	0.189	0.173	0.146
Fair	0.680	–	–	0.667	0.674	0.698
Poor	0.148	–	–	0.141	0.149	0.155
East	0.602	0.610	0.588	0.621	0.612	0.580
Urban	0.472	0.412	0.629	0.473	0.456	0.412
	Region		Residence		Economic Status	
	East	West	Urban	Rural	Rich	Poor
Observations	30,525	20,149	23,909	26,765	16,485	16,548
Male	0.477	0.476	0.479	0.475	0.507	0.463
Age						
65–79	0.267	0.271	0.249	0.286	0.398	0.374
80–89	0.339	0.376	0.380	0.329	0.281	0.286
90–99	0.261	0.235	0.254	0.247	0.208	0.219
100+	0.125	0.111	0.112	0.126	0.102	0.110
Han	0.917	0.971	0.957	0.921	0.952	0.927
Education						
Illiterate	0.559	0.567	0.483	0.633	0.486	0.602
Primary	0.318	0.312	0.335	0.299	0.340	0.315
Middle	0.119	0.117	0.178	0.065	0.171	0.080
White collar	0.094	0.098	0.162	0.037	0.148	0.051
Living arrangement						
Alone	0.147	0.132	0.129	0.152	0.078	0.118
Institution	0.031	0.047	0.060	0.017	0.019	0.023

With spouse	0.184	0.185	0.185	0.183	0.282	0.181
With children	0.473	0.491	0.459	0.500	0.452	0.482
With S & C	0.133	0.115	0.133	0.119	0.131	0.168
With others	0.032	0.030	0.033	0.029	0.037	0.028
Child paying frequent visits	0.823	0.820	0.798	0.843	0.873	0.841
Sibling paying frequent visits	0.295	0.286	0.261	0.319	0.340	0.325
# Chronic conditions	0.465	0.467	0.560	0.381	0.533	0.464
# ADLs	0.386	0.387	0.451	0.329	0.333	0.338
Perceived economic status						
Rich	0.170	0.168	0.201	0.144	0.248	0.101
Fair	0.696	0.655	0.676	0.683	0.676	0.687
Poor	0.132	0.174	0.120	0.171	0.075	0.210
East	–	–	0.613	0.593	0.602	0.605
Urban	0.480	0.459	–	–	0.464	0.435

Comparing the subsamples, there are no significant differences between eastern and central/western residents except that people were more likely to feel poor in central/western areas than their eastern counterparts.

The disparities between urban and rural residents are shown in nearly all aspects. Urban people had higher educational achievements with more decent jobs. Urban elders also had better living arrangements in that they were less likely to live alone than rural elders. And urban people felt much richer but had worse health conditions in that they had more chronic conditions and ADLs.

The differences between rich and poor show a very similar pattern as those between urban and rural except that rich people had better social network with more frequent visits by children and siblings. It is also interesting to find that about 68 % of both the rich and the poor tended to report that they were economically fair.

Empirical Strategy

We estimate the effects of government involvement in the economy on life satisfaction using Ordered Probit regressions. We relate the individuals' life satisfaction to the government involvement in the economy measured by the percentage of government consumption to GDP, the percentage of capital formation to GDP, and per capita government expenditure on public health. In Bjørnskov et al. (2007), social trust, openness to trade, the investment price are included as additional controls in the estimation regression. Since we examine the same question within China, the above variables indicating national differences are not included.

We analyze the whole sample and its subsamples by their geographic location, residence, and economic status. At the same time, we also control for individuals' characteristics and take advantage of longitudinal data to account for the time variation in the macroeconomic variables. We run an ordered probit model as follows

$$\begin{aligned} Satis_{ist} &= \alpha GDP_{st} + \beta GovCon_{st} + \gamma CapForm_{st} + \delta MedExp_{st} \\ &+ \phi Individual_{ist} + \eta_s + \theta_t + e_{ist} \end{aligned} \tag{7.1}$$

where $Satis_{ist}$ is the utility of individual, i, living in province, s, in year, t. *GovCon* represents the percentage of government consumption to GDP, *CapForm* is the percentage of capital formation to GDP, and *MedExp* is per capita government expenditure on public health. $Individual_{ist}$ refers to a vector of individual characteristics of our respondents that have been found in the previous literature to be correlated with individual life satisfaction, including gender, age, ethnicity, education, whether a white collar or not before retirement, living arrangement, social network, health conditions, and self-rated economic status. Then we also have the usual η_s, a dummy variable for residence (province), θ_t, a dummy variable for each wave of the survey and e_{ist}, an error term. We will run the estimation on the full sample, on eastern and central/western subsamples, urban and rural subsamples, and subsamples by economic status, respectively.

Results

To investigate the impact of government size on individual life satisfaction, we run ordered Probit regressions on our government size variable, which is defined before as government consumption as a percentage of GDP, by controlling a rich set of individual variables that are widely used in the happiness literature and per capita GDP.

In Table 7.4 we run the regressions for the whole sample from 1998 to 2008, which results in the estimates in the columns (1)–(4). First, after controlling for individual characteristics, real GDP per capita is negative but mostly insignificant across the board. Interestingly as we expected above, provincial governments' per capita medical expenditure has a highly significantly positive impact on these elders' life satisfaction, and the magnitudes of coefficient estimates are quite consistent across different specifications. Second, in regards to our government size variable, it has a significantly negative effect on these elders. Although the rate of capital formation has a positive impact on life satisfaction but its coefficient becomes insignificant after government size is included. Third, when we restrict our analysis to the short time period of 2002–2008 in which we have individual income variables, most of the story fortunately remains. GDP per capita is insignificantly negative, and government size is significantly negative. The only exception is that, after controlling for individual income, government medical expense does not have any significant impact, although it is still positive.

So it seems that for the whole sample in our analysis, government size does have a robust and adverse impact on elders' life satisfaction, which possibly indicates that the provincial government's activities might not be in line with elders' preferences. In the following section, we would like to explore sub-population heterogeneity by considering the potential difference between urban and rural residents, eastern and western residents, and the rich and the poor.

Although the relationships between individual life satisfaction and individual characteristics are not our focus, it is important to check whether these relationships are consistent with the evidence found in the literature. From this perspective, Chinese do not look quite different from the rest of the world. First, living with someone is significantly positively correlated with higher levels of life satisfaction, compared with living alone. Second, the more educated the individual is, the more satisfied she is with her life. Third, respondents who are frequently visited by either their children or their siblings report higher levels of satisfaction than those who are not. Fourth, income does buy happiness. Households who belong to the top 3 income quartiles report higher levels of satisfaction than those in the bottom quartile. Besides, feeling richer also brings more satisfaction to these elders.

Table 7.4 GDP, government size and life satisfaction – The whole sample

	1998–2008 (no income variables)				2002–2008 (w/income variables)			
	(1)	(2)	(3)	(4)	(5)	(6)	(7)	(8)
Variables	Base	Govt size	Capital	All	Base	Govt size	Capital	All
Real GDP per capita	−0.0140*	−0.00348	−0.00845	−0.00289	−0.0147	−0.00172	−0.0118	−0.00157
	(0.00769)	(0.00858)	(0.00816)	(0.00862)	(0.0123)	(0.0135)	(0.0126)	(0.0135)
Gov't medical expense	0.00215***	0.00214***	0.00206***	0.00211***	0.000467	0.000673	0.000488	0.000688
	(0.000460)	(0.000459)	(0.000460)	(0.000461)	(0.000663)	(0.000667)	(0.000663)	(0.000668)
Gov't size		−0.0119***		−0.0103**		−0.0144**		−0.0162**
		(0.00418)		(0.00496)		(0.00602)		(0.00754)
Capital formation rate			0.00249**	0.000919			0.00177	−0.000916
			(0.00123)	(0.00147)			(0.00174)	(0.00218)
Male	−0.0544***	−0.0545***	−0.0543***	−0.0544***	−0.0394***	−0.0396***	−0.0395***	−0.0396***
	(0.0116)	(0.0116)	(0.0116)	(0.0116)	(0.0144)	(0.0144)	(0.0144)	(0.0144)
Live institutionally	0.614***	0.612***	0.614***	0.612***	0.610***	0.609***	0.610***	0.609***
	(0.0283)	(0.0284)	(0.0283)	(0.0284)	(0.0502)	(0.0502)	(0.0502)	(0.0502)
Live w/spouse	0.266***	0.267***	0.267***	0.267***	0.181***	0.181***	0.182***	0.181***
	(0.0186)	(0.0186)	(0.0187)	(0.0187)	(0.0250)	(0.0250)	(0.0250)	(0.0250)
Live w/child	0.425***	0.425***	0.425***	0.425***	0.261***	0.261***	0.262***	0.261***
	(0.0155)	(0.0155)	(0.0155)	(0.0155)	(0.0227)	(0.0227)	(0.0227)	(0.0227)
Live w/child & spouse	0.346***	0.346***	0.346***	0.346***	0.226***	0.226***	0.227***	0.226***
	(0.0200)	(0.0200)	(0.0200)	(0.0200)	(0.0265)	(0.0265)	(0.0265)	(0.0265)
Live w/other(s)	0.324***	0.325***	0.325***	0.326***	0.231***	0.234***	0.233***	0.233***
	(0.0317)	(0.0317)	(0.0317)	(0.0317)	(0.0410)	(0.0410)	(0.0410)	(0.0410)
Age group 3	0.0667***	0.0665***	0.0667***	0.0665***	0.0481***	0.0478***	0.0482***	0.0477***
	(0.0143)	(0.0143)	(0.0143)	(0.0143)	(0.0163)	(0.0163)	(0.0163)	(0.0163)
Age group 4	0.178***	0.178***	0.178***	0.178***	0.158***	0.158***	0.158***	0.158***
	(0.0162)	(0.0162)	(0.0162)	(0.0162)	(0.0192)	(0.0192)	(0.0192)	(0.0192)

Age group 5	0.304***	0.304***	0.304***	0.304***	0.287***	0.287***	0.287***	0.287***
	(0.0199)	(0.0199)	(0.0199)	(0.0199)	(0.0243)	(0.0243)	(0.0243)	(0.0243)
Urban (=1)	0.155***	0.155***	0.155***	0.155***	0.0608***	0.0603***	0.0608***	0.0603***
	(0.0107)	(0.0107)	(0.0107)	(0.0107)	(0.0138)	(0.0138)	(0.0138)	(0.0138)
Han ethnicity (=1)	−0.0775***	−0.0777***	−0.0770***	−0.0775***	−0.120***	−0.120***	−0.120***	−0.120***
	(0.0215)	(0.0215)	(0.0215)	(0.0215)	(0.0273)	(0.0273)	(0.0273)	(0.0273)
Primary education	0.0852***	0.0854***	0.0850***	0.0853***	0.0322**	0.0327**	0.0323**	0.0327**
	(0.0124)	(0.0124)	(0.0124)	(0.0124)	(0.0155)	(0.0155)	(0.0155)	(0.0155)
Secondary education	0.180***	0.180***	0.179***	0.180***	0.0578**	0.0581**	0.0575**	0.0583**
	(0.0200)	(0.0200)	(0.0200)	(0.0200)	(0.0251)	(0.0251)	(0.0251)	(0.0251)
White collar (=1)	0.273***	0.273***	0.273***	0.273***	0.115***	0.115***	0.115***	0.115***
	(0.0208)	(0.0208)	(0.0208)	(0.0208)	(0.0261)	(0.0260)	(0.0260)	(0.0260)
Frequently visited by child (=1)	0.182***	0.182***	0.182***	0.182***	0.118***	0.118***	0.118***	0.118***
	(0.0136)	(0.0136)	(0.0136)	(0.0136)	(0.0186)	(0.0186)	(0.0186)	(0.0186)
Frequently visited by sibling (=1)	0.0776***	0.0776***	0.0775***	0.0776***	0.0306**	0.0306**	0.0306**	0.0306**
	(0.0117)	(0.0117)	(0.0117)	(0.0117)	(0.0144)	(0.0144)	(0.0144)	(0.0144)
Chronic score	−0.0792***	−0.0790***	−0.0793***	−0.0790***	−0.0680***	−0.0681***	−0.0680***	−0.0680***
	(0.00696)	(0.00696)	(0.00696)	(0.00696)	(0.00855)	(0.00854)	(0.00854)	(0.00855)
Adl score	−0.0563***	−0.0564***	−0.0563***	−0.0564***	−0.0519***	−0.0522***	−0.0520***	−0.0522***
	(0.00530)	(0.00530)	(0.00530)	(0.00530)	(0.00729)	(0.00729)	(0.00729)	(0.00729)
2nd income quartile					0.141***	0.142***	0.141***	0.142***
					(0.0178)	(0.0178)	(0.0178)	(0.0178)
3rd income quartile					0.204***	0.205***	0.204***	0.205***
					(0.0188)	(0.0188)	(0.0188)	(0.0188)
4th income quartile					0.271***	0.271***	0.270***	0.272***
					(0.0206)	(0.0206)	(0.0206)	(0.0206)

(continued)

Table 7.4 (continued)

	1998–2008 (no income variables)				2002–2008 (w/income variables)			
	(1)	(2)	(3)	(4)	(5)	(6)	(7)	(8)
Variables	Base	Govt size	Capital	All	Base	Govt size	Capital	All
Feeling rich (=1)					1.569***	1.568***	1.569***	1.568***
					(0.0265)	(0.0265)	(0.0265)	(0.0265)
Feeling fair (=1)					0.893***	0.892***	0.893***	0.892***
					(0.0212)	(0.0212)	(0.0212)	(0.0212)
Wave_2000	−0.0977***	−0.0833***	−0.0954***	−0.0844***				
	(0.0180)	(0.0188)	(0.0180)	(0.0189)				
Wave_2002	−0.293***	−0.268***	−0.293***	−0.271***	−0.0439	0.0345	−0.0152	0.0296
	(0.0170)	(0.0191)	(0.0170)	(0.0200)	(0.0370)	(0.0503)	(0.0465)	(0.0511)
Wave_2005	−0.264***	−0.268***	−0.286***	−0.276***	0.0190	0.0594*	0.0331	0.0572*
	(0.0211)	(0.0212)	(0.0239)	(0.0244)	(0.0276)	(0.0331)	(0.0309)	(0.0333)
Wave_2008	−0.363***	−0.394***	−0.402***	−0.404***				
	(0.0300)	(0.0322)	(0.0358)	(0.0358)				
Province dummies	Yes	Yes	Yes	Yes	Yes	Yes	Yes	Yes
Observations	50,403	50,403	50,403	50,403	32,887	32,887	32,887	32,887

(1) Heteroskedastic- robust standard errors in parentheses. *** $p < 0.01$, ** $p < 0.05$, * $p < 0.1$
(2) Age groups are also controlled. Time dummies and province dummies are also included
(3) The default group for Living Arrangements is living alone. The default group for Primary and Secondary Education is illiterate. The default group for income quartiles is the bottom quartile

Finally, having more chronic diseases or having more difficulties in daily lives is negatively correlated with life satisfaction.

Urban Versus Rural Residents

To further investigate the potential heterogeneity between urban and rural residents, in Table 7.5 we report our regression results for the urban and rural subsamples separately.

First, real GDP per capita enters the urban regression positively but statistically it is either insignificant or only marginally significant (columns (1), (2), (5) and (6)). In contrast it is significantly negative in the rural subsample. Second, government size is robustly significantly negative only in the urban subsample, and it is positive but insignificant for rural residents. Third, government medical expense only has a significantly positive impact on rural elders.

Finally, in terms of individual characteristics, there are a few differences between the urban and rural subsamples, in particular when income variables are controlled for. There seems to be no gender difference, after controlling for income variables, among urban residents, but rural males are significantly more unsatisfied with their lives than rural females. After controlling for incomes, education loses significance and becomes less significant in the rural sample than in the urban sample. Results for the other characteristics are quite similar to the results for the whole sample in Table 7.4.

East Versus West

Eastern China has been enjoying a more rapid growth than western China over the past 30 years. It is interesting to see whether residents in a more developed area have different preferences over the government activities than those in the area that is lagging behind.

In Table 7.6 it is interesting to note that real GDP per capita is robustly negatively correlated with individual life satisfaction in the western area, whether income variables are controlled for or not, while it is first insignificant in the eastern area but becomes significantly positive after household income is controlled for. More interestingly government size has distinctly different impacts in these two areas. It seems that government activities are more in line with western residents but are not lined up with eastern residents. One possibility could be that western governments, due to the region's low income level and correspondingly lower fiscal revenues, are getting more transfers from the central government, which ended up improving their residents' welfare, while residents in more developed eastern provinces have to look after themselves. The negative impact of capital formation rate in eastern area seems to corroborate with this conjecture because more

Table 7.5 GDP, government size and life satisfaction – Urban vs. rural

	1998–2008 (no income variables)				2002–2008 (w/income variables)			
	(1)	(2)	(3)	(4)	(5)	(6)	(7)	(8)
	Urban		Rural		Urban		Rural	
Variables	Base	Govt size	Base	Govt size	Base	Govt size	Base	Govt size
Real GDP per capita	0.00450	0.0214*	−0.0249**	−0.0347**	0.0150	0.0337*	−0.0427**	−0.0559***
	(0.0104)	(0.0113)	(0.0118)	(0.0136)	(0.0170)	(0.0179)	(0.0180)	(0.0208)
Gov't medical expense	0.000951*	0.00110*	0.00390***	0.00419***	−0.00126	−0.000495	0.00333***	0.00350***
	(0.000562)	(0.000564)	(0.000899)	(0.000922)	(0.000814)	(0.000843)	(0.00122)	(0.00124)
Gov't size		−0.0178***		0.00370		−0.0304***		0.00910
		(0.00667)		(0.00762)		(0.0101)		(0.0117)
Capital formation rate		0.00255		−0.00233		−0.000832		−0.00141
		(0.00194)		(0.00230)		(0.00284)		(0.00350)
Male	−0.0305*	−0.0303*	−0.0756***	−0.0757***	−0.0187	−0.0187	−0.0530***	−0.0528***
	(0.0169)	(0.0169)	(0.0160)	(0.0160)	(0.0216)	(0.0216)	(0.0195)	(0.0195)
Live institutionally	0.564***	0.560***	0.694***	0.694***	0.608***	0.606***	0.570***	0.571***
	(0.0350)	(0.0351)	(0.0532)	(0.0532)	(0.0622)	(0.0622)	(0.0892)	(0.0893)
Live w/spouse	0.269***	0.271***	0.259***	0.259***	0.156***	0.155***	0.198***	0.197***
	(0.0278)	(0.0278)	(0.0253)	(0.0253)	(0.0381)	(0.0381)	(0.0333)	(0.0334)
Live w/child	0.391***	0.391***	0.452***	0.451***	0.242***	0.241***	0.275***	0.274***
	(0.0235)	(0.0235)	(0.0208)	(0.0208)	(0.0347)	(0.0347)	(0.0302)	(0.0303)
Live w/child & spouse	0.290***	0.290***	0.399***	0.398***	0.170***	0.168***	0.276***	0.275***
	(0.0296)	(0.0296)	(0.0273)	(0.0273)	(0.0402)	(0.0403)	(0.0355)	(0.0355)
Live w/other(s)	0.324***	0.325***	0.324***	0.322***	0.256***	0.258***	0.208***	0.206***
	(0.0453)	(0.0452)	(0.0449)	(0.0449)	(0.0600)	(0.0601)	(0.0564)	(0.0564)
Age group 3	0.0911***	0.0913***	0.0451**	0.0453**	0.0580**	0.0567**	0.0452**	0.0453**
	(0.0213)	(0.0213)	(0.0194)	(0.0194)	(0.0245)	(0.0245)	(0.0220)	(0.0220)

Age group 4	0.183***	0.184***	0.173***	0.173***	0.147***	0.146***	0.178***	0.178***
	(0.0241)	(0.0241)	(0.0222)	(0.0222)	(0.0289)	(0.0289)	(0.0260)	(0.0260)
Age group 5	0.370***	0.368***	0.256***	0.257***	0.329***	0.326***	0.263***	0.263***
	(0.0302)	(0.0302)	(0.0267)	(0.0267)	(0.0368)	(0.0368)	(0.0328)	(0.0328)
Han ethnicity (=1)	−0.137***	−0.136***	−0.0462*	−0.0465*	−0.120**	−0.120**	−0.135***	−0.135***
	(0.0372)	(0.0372)	(0.0268)	(0.0268)	(0.0484)	(0.0485)	(0.0337)	(0.0337)
Primary education	0.0852***	0.0852***	0.0886***	0.0885***	0.0353	0.0362	0.0308	0.0303
	(0.0179)	(0.0179)	(0.0172)	(0.0172)	(0.0232)	(0.0232)	(0.0209)	(0.0209)
Secondary education	0.178***	0.178***	0.192***	0.192***	0.0573*	0.0575*	0.0499	0.0494
	(0.0258)	(0.0258)	(0.0320)	(0.0320)	(0.0331)	(0.0331)	(0.0394)	(0.0394)
White collar (=1)	0.283***	0.283***	0.212***	0.211***	0.112***	0.110***	0.0846*	0.0842*
	(0.0245)	(0.0245)	(0.0399)	(0.0399)	(0.0311)	(0.0310)	(0.0482)	(0.0482)
Frequently visited by child (=1)	0.131***	0.131***	0.238***	0.238***	0.0681**	0.0677**	0.165***	0.165***
	(0.0190)	(0.0190)	(0.0195)	(0.0195)	(0.0266)	(0.0266)	(0.0260)	(0.0260)
Frequently visited by sibling (=1)	0.0826***	0.0825***	0.0704***	0.0705***	0.0494**	0.0493**	0.0162	0.0162
	(0.0176)	(0.0176)	(0.0158)	(0.0158)	(0.0223)	(0.0223)	(0.0190)	(0.0190)
Chronic score	−0.0729***	−0.0728***	−0.0831***	−0.0832***	−0.0651***	−0.0652***	−0.0705***	−0.0704***
	(0.00915)	(0.00915)	(0.0107)	(0.0107)	(0.0113)	(0.0113)	(0.0130)	(0.0130)
Adl score	−0.0487***	−0.0489***	−0.0667***	−0.0667***	−0.0447***	−0.0452***	−0.0643***	−0.0641***
	(0.00739)	(0.00739)	(0.00758)	(0.00758)	(0.0101)	(0.0101)	(0.0105)	(0.0105)
2nd income quartile					0.112***	0.113***	0.160***	0.160***
					(0.0340)	(0.0340)	(0.0214)	(0.0214)
3rd income quartile					0.194***	0.196***	0.241***	0.241***
					(0.0317)	(0.0317)	(0.0248)	(0.0248)
4th income quartile					0.321***	0.323***	0.210***	0.209***
					(0.0326)	(0.0326)	(0.0287)	(0.0287)
Feeling rich (=1)					1.541***	1.541***	1.571***	1.572***
					(0.0412)	(0.0413)	(0.0353)	(0.0353)

(continued)

Table 7.5 (continued)

	1998–2008 (no income variables)				2002–2008 (w/income variables)			
	(1)	(2)	(3)	(4)	(5)	(6)	(7)	(8)
	Urban		Rural		Urban		Rural	
Variables	Base	Govt size	Base	Govt size	Base	Govt size	Base	Govt size
Feeling fair (=1)					0.857***	0.855***	0.914***	0.915***
					(0.0349)	(0.0350)	(0.0269)	(0.0269)
Wave_2000	−0.109***	−0.0854***	−0.0930***	−0.0993***				
	(0.0255)	(0.0266)	(0.0268)	(0.0280)				
Wave_2002	−0.293***	−0.255***	−0.305***	−0.314***	−0.0202	0.122*	−0.0154	−0.0832
	(0.0261)	(0.0297)	(0.0229)	(0.0279)	(0.0513)	(0.0707)	(0.0619)	(0.0790)
Wave_2005	−0.300***	−0.325***	−0.257***	−0.236***	0.00984	0.0856*	0.0721	0.0411
	(0.0321)	(0.0365)	(0.0299)	(0.0341)	(0.0371)	(0.0455)	(0.0483)	(0.0543)
Wave_2008	−0.374***	−0.455***	−0.399***	−0.358***				
	(0.0416)	(0.0497)	(0.0535)	(0.0589)				
Province dummies	Yes	Yes	Yes	Yes	Yes	Yes	Yes	Yes
Observations	23,784	23,784	26,619	26,619	14,769	14,769	18,118	18,118

(1) Heteroskedastic- robust standard errors in parentheses. *** $p < 0.01$, ** $p < 0.05$, * $p < 0.1$

(2) Age groups are also controlled. Time dummies and province dummies are also included

(3) The default group for Living Arrangements is living alone. The default group for Primary and Secondary Education is illiterate. The default group for income quartiles is the bottom quartile

Table 7.6 GDP, government size and life satisfaction – East vs. West

	1998–2008 (no income variables)				2002–2008 (w/income variables)			
	(1)	(2)	(3)	(4)	(5)	(6)	(7)	(8)
	East		West		East		West	
Variables	Base	Gov't size	Base	Govt size	Base	Govt size	Base	Govt size
Real GDP per capita	−0.0163*	0.00548	−0.0449**	−0.117***	−0.00377	0.0367**	−0.134***	−0.181***
	(0.00941)	(0.0113)	(0.0175)	(0.0211)	(0.0150)	(0.0172)	(0.0280)	(0.0327)
Gov't medical expense	0.00205***	0.00249***	0.00391***	0.00412***	−0.000267	0.000386	0.0228***	0.0220***
	(0.000520)	(0.000530)	(0.00122)	(0.00122)	(0.000703)	(0.000708)	(0.00359)	(0.00359)
Gov't size		−0.0610***		0.0342***		−0.0797***		0.0496***
		(0.00777)		(0.00748)		(0.0107)		(0.0133)
Capital formation rate		−0.0128***		0.0129***		−0.0177***		0.00503
		(0.00249)		(0.00268)		(0.00363)		(0.00413)
Male	−0.0611***	−0.0619***	−0.0438**	−0.0423**	−0.0310*	−0.0315*	−0.0529**	−0.0520**
	(0.0151)	(0.0151)	(0.0181)	(0.0181)	(0.0186)	(0.0186)	(0.0229)	(0.0229)
Live institutionally	0.601***	0.590***	0.630***	0.634***	0.567***	0.572***	0.682***	0.690***
	(0.0396)	(0.0397)	(0.0418)	(0.0419)	(0.0642)	(0.0642)	(0.0805)	(0.0809)
Live w/spouse	0.239***	0.240***	0.310***	0.308***	0.148***	0.141***	0.237***	0.237***
	(0.0238)	(0.0238)	(0.0300)	(0.0300)	(0.0316)	(0.0316)	(0.0409)	(0.0409)
Live w/child	0.418***	0.419***	0.437***	0.436***	0.235***	0.231***	0.299***	0.297***
	(0.0197)	(0.0197)	(0.0252)	(0.0252)	(0.0285)	(0.0285)	(0.0375)	(0.0375)
Live w/child & spouse	0.299***	0.299***	0.429***	0.429***	0.163***	0.157***	0.337***	0.337***
	(0.0252)	(0.0252)	(0.0330)	(0.0330)	(0.0333)	(0.0333)	(0.0440)	(0.0439)
Live w/other(s)	0.324***	0.328***	0.325***	0.328***	0.195***	0.199***	0.294***	0.302***
	(0.0405)	(0.0404)	(0.0511)	(0.0509)	(0.0533)	(0.0535)	(0.0641)	(0.0640)
Age group 3	0.0252	0.0240	0.130***	0.129***	0.0350*	0.0327	0.0752***	0.0767***
	(0.0185)	(0.0184)	(0.0227)	(0.0227)	(0.0210)	(0.0210)	(0.0260)	(0.0260)

(continued)

Table 7.6 (continued)

	1998–2008 (no income variables)				2002–2008 (w/income variables)			
	(1)	(2)	(3)	(4)	(5)	(6)	(7)	(8)
	East		West		East		West	
Variables	Base	Gov't size	Base	Govt size	Base	Govt size	Base	Govt size
Age group 4	0.142***	0.140***	0.237***	0.233***	0.129***	0.127***	0.217***	0.216***
	(0.0206)	(0.0206)	(0.0265)	(0.0265)	(0.0242)	(0.0242)	(0.0320)	(0.0319)
Age group 5	0.259***	0.259***	0.376***	0.371***	0.274***	0.277***	0.320***	0.322***
	(0.0252)	(0.0252)	(0.0325)	(0.0325)	(0.0309)	(0.0309)	(0.0398)	(0.0398)
Urban (=1)	0.140***	0.142***	0.172***	0.173***	0.0637***	0.0602***	0.0565**	0.0573**
	(0.0138)	(0.0138)	(0.0172)	(0.0172)	(0.0176)	(0.0176)	(0.0224)	(0.0225)
Han ethnicity (=1)	−0.0638***	−0.0654***	−0.116**	−0.121**	−0.167***	−0.168***	−0.0149	−0.0171
	(0.0239)	(0.0239)	(0.0483)	(0.0485)	(0.0303)	(0.0304)	(0.0640)	(0.0643)
Primary education	0.0688***	0.0700***	0.113***	0.110***	0.0224	0.0249	0.0511**	0.0498**
	(0.0161)	(0.0162)	(0.0194)	(0.0194)	(0.0201)	(0.0201)	(0.0244)	(0.0244)
Secondary education	0.181***	0.185***	0.183***	0.179***	0.0509	0.0540*	0.0786**	0.0755*
	(0.0262)	(0.0262)	(0.0312)	(0.0313)	(0.0326)	(0.0326)	(0.0398)	(0.0399)
White collar (=1)	0.265***	0.267***	0.279***	0.281***	0.117***	0.115***	0.113***	0.113***
	(0.0268)	(0.0268)	(0.0331)	(0.0332)	(0.0330)	(0.0330)	(0.0427)	(0.0428)
Frequently visited by child (=1)	0.181***	0.179***	0.186***	0.189***	0.152***	0.151***	0.0659**	0.0668**
	(0.0175)	(0.0175)	(0.0218)	(0.0218)	(0.0236)	(0.0237)	(0.0300)	(0.0300)
Frequently visited by sibling (=1)	0.0652***	0.0646***	0.101***	0.100***	0.0338*	0.0341*	0.0253	0.0247
	(0.0151)	(0.0151)	(0.0187)	(0.0187)	(0.0186)	(0.0186)	(0.0228)	(0.0228)
Chronic score	−0.0753***	−0.0728***	−0.0830***	−0.0834***	−0.0668***	−0.0645***	−0.0697***	−0.0679***
	(0.00893)	(0.00894)	(0.0112)	(0.0112)	(0.0110)	(0.0110)	(0.0136)	(0.0137)
Adl score	−0.0498***	−0.0503***	−0.0690***	−0.0683***	−0.0435***	−0.0445***	−0.0674***	−0.0674***
	(0.00665)	(0.00665)	(0.00879)	(0.00880)	(0.00909)	(0.00909)	(0.0123)	(0.0123)

2nd income quartile					0.172***	0.175***	0.123***	0.128***
					(0.0248)	(0.0248)	(0.0263)	(0.0263)
3rd income quartile					0.263***	0.267***	0.144***	0.150***
					(0.0254)	(0.0254)	(0.0291)	(0.0291)
4th income quartile					0.309***	0.320***	0.235***	0.240***
					(0.0270)	(0.0271)	(0.0331)	(0.0331)
Feeling rich (=1)					1.617***	1.611***	1.519***	1.517***
					(0.0354)	(0.0354)	(0.0406)	(0.0406)
Feeling fair (=1)					0.927***	0.921***	0.858***	0.859***
					(0.0289)	(0.0289)	(0.0314)	(0.0314)
Wave_2000	−0.133***	−0.0815***	−0.0445	−0.0853***	N.A.	N.A.	N.A.	N.A.
	(0.0233)	(0.0245)	(0.0286)	(0.0301)				
Wave_2002	−0.288***	−0.166***	−0.303***	−0.379***	−0.0429	0.134**	0.738***	0.544***
	(0.0221)	(0.0272)	(0.0272)	(0.0318)	(0.0453)	(0.0663)	(0.148)	(0.155)
Wave_2005	−0.246***	−0.162***	−0.267***	−0.298***	0.0270	0.140***	0.733***	0.630***
	(0.0289)	(0.0369)	(0.0349)	(0.0358)	(0.0309)	(0.0389)	(0.130)	(0.132)
Wave_2008	−0.337***	−0.328***	−0.386***	−0.386***	Default	Default	Default	Default
	(0.0374)	(0.0475)	(0.0735)	(0.0742)				
Province dummies	Yes	Yes	Yes	Yes	Yes	Yes	Yes	Yes
Observations	30,379	30,379	20,024	20,024	19,880	19,880	13,007	13,007

(1) Heteroskedastic- robust standard errors in parentheses. *** $p < 0.01$, ** $p < 0.05$, * $p < 0.1$

(2) Age groups are also controlled. Time dummies and province dummies are also included

(3) The default group for Living Arrangements is living alone. The default group for Primary and Secondary Education is illiterate. The default group for income quartiles is the bottom quartile

developed provincial governments have economic growth as their top priority (Li and Zhou 2005).

The good news is that government medical expense has a significantly positive impact on western residents, even after controlling for all income variables.

Rich Versus Poor

In theory the rich and the poor may have different preferences over government activities. In Table 7.7 we carry out separate regressions for the rich and the poor. Please note that we have income information for each household only after 2000. Interestingly government size has a significantly negative impact on life satisfaction of the rich but have no significant impacts on the poor. Real GDP per capita has a mostly positive impact on the rich's life satisfaction while it brings adverse impacts to the poor. The good news for the poor is that the per capita government medical spending brings positive benefits to them.

Conclusions

Why are Chinese lagging behind in their reported levels of life satisfaction during a period of spectacular economic growth? We endeavor to investigate one of the potential factors: government size. We apply ordered Probit regressions to a unique data set of five rounds of surveys on Chinese elders between 1998 and 2008, which interviews over 10,000 individuals who are located in 22 provinces. Controlling for individual characteristics commonly found to be correlated with individual life satisfaction across the world, provincial GDP per capita, government size and medical expense are included in the regressions to investigate their impacts.

In general we find that government size is detrimental to elders' life satisfaction, the coefficient of which is quite significant and robust across different specifications. It seems to indicate that for the general population of elders in China, more government activities are not in line with their elder residents' preferences, which might be, to a large extent, due to the fact that local governments usually put priority on economic growth mainly measured by GDP. Furthermore, we find very interesting results by looking at subpopulation heterogeneities. One of them is that the adverse impact of government size seems to be concentrated on richer residents and residents who are located in more developed regions, whether they being urban or eastern. In contrast we find insignificantly positive impacts for rural and poor residents and even significantly positive impact for western (less developed) residents, which is possibly due to the dependence on social welfare of these regions lagging behind the national average.

Another interesting finding is about the relationship between real GDP per capita and life satisfaction. Although GDP is insignificantly negative for the whole

Table 7.7 GDP, government size and life satisfaction – Rich vs. poor

	Rich				Poor			
	(1)	(2)	(3)	(4)	(5)	(6)	(7)	(8)
Variables	Base	Govt size	Capital	All	Base	Govt size	Capital	All
Real GDP per capita	0.0237	0.0428**	0.0304*	0.0428**	−0.0698***	−0.0862***	−0.0775***	−0.0832***
	(0.0159)	(0.0168)	(0.0162)	(0.0168)	(0.0199)	(0.0231)	(0.0203)	(0.0234)
Gov't medical expense	−0.00109	−0.000394	−0.000926	−0.000395	0.00379***	0.00394***	0.00413***	0.00412***
	(0.000784)	(0.000810)	(0.000789)	(0.000810)	(0.00137)	(0.00137)	(0.00139)	(0.00139)
Gov't size		−0.0282***		−0.0280***		0.0135		0.00629
		(0.00811)		(0.00985)		(0.00939)		(0.0123)
Capital formation rate			0.00448*	9.71e-05			−0.00458*	−0.00347
			(0.00232)	(0.00282)			(0.00277)	(0.00363)
Male	−0.0643***	−0.0648***	−0.0645***	−0.0648***	−0.0155	−0.0157	−0.0157	−0.0157
	(0.0199)	(0.0199)	(0.0199)	(0.0199)	(0.0211)	(0.0211)	(0.0211)	(0.0211)
Live institutionally	0.380***	0.378***	0.380***	0.378***	0.889***	0.891***	0.891***	0.891***
	(0.0683)	(0.0683)	(0.0683)	(0.0683)	(0.0736)	(0.0736)	(0.0735)	(0.0736)
Live w/spouse	0.157***	0.157***	0.159***	0.157***	0.187***	0.187***	0.184***	0.185***
	(0.0374)	(0.0374)	(0.0374)	(0.0374)	(0.0340)	(0.0340)	(0.0341)	(0.0341)
Live w/child	0.211***	0.209***	0.212***	0.209***	0.294***	0.293***	0.292***	0.292***
	(0.0343)	(0.0343)	(0.0343)	(0.0343)	(0.0307)	(0.0307)	(0.0308)	(0.0308)
Live w/child & spouse	0.142***	0.140***	0.143***	0.140***	0.300***	0.299***	0.298***	0.298***
	(0.0390)	(0.0390)	(0.0390)	(0.0391)	(0.0368)	(0.0368)	(0.0368)	(0.0368)
Live w/other(s)	0.187***	0.188***	0.191***	0.188***	0.274***	0.271***	0.270***	0.269***
	(0.0562)	(0.0562)	(0.0562)	(0.0563)	(0.0611)	(0.0611)	(0.0612)	(0.0612)
Age group 3	0.0529**	0.0522**	0.0528**	0.0522**	0.0427*	0.0429*	0.0423*	0.0425*
	(0.0229)	(0.0229)	(0.0229)	(0.0229)	(0.0234)	(0.0234)	(0.0234)	(0.0234)
Age group 4	0.134***	0.134***	0.133***	0.134***	0.194***	0.194***	0.194***	0.194***
	(0.0270)	(0.0271)	(0.0270)	(0.0271)	(0.0276)	(0.0276)	(0.0276)	(0.0276)

(continued)

Table 7.7 (continued)

	Rich				Poor			
	(1)	(2)	(3)	(4)	(5)	(6)	(7)	(8)
Variables	Base	Govt size	Capital	All	Base	Govt size	Capital	All
Age group 5	0.300***	0.299***	0.298***	0.299***	0.277***	0.277***	0.277***	0.277***
	(0.0340)	(0.0340)	(0.0340)	(0.0340)	(0.0351)	(0.0351)	(0.0351)	(0.0351)
Urban (=1)	0.0810***	0.0814***	0.0812***	0.0814***	0.0444**	0.0454**	0.0444**	0.0449**
	(0.0188)	(0.0188)	(0.0188)	(0.0188)	(0.0208)	(0.0208)	(0.0208)	(0.0208)
Han ethnicity (=1)	−0.0243	−0.0234	−0.0227	−0.0234	−0.197***	−0.197***	−0.197***	−0.197***
	(0.0438)	(0.0438)	(0.0438)	(0.0438)	(0.0357)	(0.0357)	(0.0357)	(0.0357)
Primary education	0.0518**	0.0527**	0.0518**	0.0526**	0.0129	0.0126	0.0125	0.0124
	(0.0216)	(0.0216)	(0.0216)	(0.0216)	(0.0223)	(0.0223)	(0.0223)	(0.0223)
Secondary education	0.0574*	0.0577*	0.0563*	0.0576*	0.0683	0.0683	0.0686	0.0685
	(0.0315)	(0.0315)	(0.0315)	(0.0315)	(0.0426)	(0.0427)	(0.0427)	(0.0427)
White collar (=1)	0.125***	0.124***	0.125***	0.124***	0.0676	0.0682	0.0672	0.0676
	(0.0301)	(0.0301)	(0.0301)	(0.0301)	(0.0545)	(0.0545)	(0.0544)	(0.0545)
Frequently visited by child (=1)	0.0934***	0.0931***	0.0936***	0.0931***	0.157***	0.157***	0.157***	0.157***
	(0.0261)	(0.0261)	(0.0261)	(0.0261)	(0.0266)	(0.0266)	(0.0266)	(0.0266)
Frequently visited by Sibling (=1)	0.0415**	0.0414**	0.0412**	0.0413**	0.0183	0.0183	0.0184	0.0184
	(0.0205)	(0.0206)	(0.0205)	(0.0206)	(0.0203)	(0.0203)	(0.0203)	(0.0203)
Chronic score	−0.0672***	−0.0669***	−0.0672***	−0.0669***	−0.0676***	−0.0671***	−0.0670***	−0.0669***
	(0.0109)	(0.0109)	(0.0109)	(0.0109)	(0.0137)	(0.0137)	(0.0137)	(0.0137)
Adl score	−0.0555***	−0.0561***	−0.0555***	−0.0561***	−0.0486***	−0.0484***	−0.0482***	−0.0482***
	(0.00975)	(0.00975)	(0.00975)	(0.00975)	(0.0110)	(0.0110)	(0.0110)	(0.0110)
2nd income quartile					0.160***	0.160***	0.160***	0.159***
					(0.0185)	(0.0185)	(0.0185)	(0.0185)

3rd income quartile	−0.0622***	−0.0628***	−0.0620***	−0.0628***				
	(0.0185)	(0.0185)	(0.0185)	(0.0185)				
Feeling rich (=1)	1.562***	1.561***	1.561***	1.561***	1.545***	1.547***	1.545***	1.546***
	(0.0462)	(0.0462)	(0.0462)	(0.0462)	(0.0379)	(0.0379)	(0.0379)	(0.0379)
Feeling fair (=1)	0.872***	0.871***	0.872***	0.871***	0.897***	0.898***	0.896***	0.897***
	(0.0426)	(0.0426)	(0.0426)	(0.0426)	(0.0247)	(0.0247)	(0.0247)	(0.0247)
Wave_2002	0.0412	0.186***	0.116*	0.186***	−0.0869	−0.159*	−0.147*	−0.166*
	(0.0483)	(0.0649)	(0.0615)	(0.0668)	(0.0695)	(0.0866)	(0.0777)	(0.0864)
Wave_2005	0.0434	0.118***	0.0811**	0.119***	0.0444	0.00959	0.0202	0.00983
	(0.0349)	(0.0421)	(0.0400)	(0.0427)	(0.0540)	(0.0600)	(0.0557)	(0.0600)
Wave_2008	Default	Default	Default	Default	Default	Default	Default	Default
Province dummies	Yes	Yes	Yes	Yes	Yes	Yes	Yes	Yes
Observations	17,014	17,014	17,014	17,014	15,873	15,873	15,873	15,873

(1) Heteroskedastic- robust standard errors in parentheses. *** $p < 0.01$, ** $p < 0.05$, * $p < 0.1$

(2) Age groups are also controlled. Time dummies and province dummies are also included

(3) The default group for Living Arrangements is living alone. The default group for Primary and Secondary Education is illiterate. The default group for income quartiles is the bottom quartile

sample, it seems to be robustly significantly negative for rural, western or poor residents. In contrast rich residents are more likely to be satisfied with life when real GDP per capita is higher. This shows evidence that GDP brings uneven benefits to the population.

Finally we acknowledge the existence of data shortcomings in this paper, in particular the lack of detailed information on inter-governmental transfers and the itemized government expenditures. As this kind of data is generally not publicly available, our analysis is best interpreted as a first attempt to measure the aggregate impact of government size on Chinese elders' life satisfaction. Therefore further research could be carried out along the line of measuring the fiscal institutions and disaggregated fiscal expenditures and then applying the same analysis on individuals' life satisfaction.[7]

References

Alesina, A., Di Tella, R., & MacCulloch, R. (2004). Inequality and happiness: Are Europeans and Americans different? *Journal of Public Economics, 88*, 2009–2042.

Bjørnskov, C., Dreher, A., & Fischer, J. A. V. (2007). The bigger the better: Evidence of the effect of government size on life satisfaction around the world. *Public Choice, 130*, 267–292.

Brockmann, H., Delhey, J., Welzel, C., & Hao Yuan. (2009). The China puzzle: Falling happiness in a rising economy. *Journal of Happiness Studies, 10*(4), 387–405.

Clark, A. E., Frijters, P., & Shields, M. A. (2008). Relative income, happiness and utility: An explanation for the Easterli-Paradox and other puzzles. *Journal of Economic Literature, 46*, 95–144.

Crabtree, S., & Wu, T. (2011). China's puzzling flat line. *Gallup Management Journal*. http://gmj.gallup.com/content/148853/china-puzzling-flat-line.aspx#1. Accessed 9 Jan 2013.

Di Tella, R., & MacCulloch, R. (2006). Some uses of happiness data in economics. *Journal of Economic Perspectives, 20*(1 Winter), 25–46.

Di Tella, R., MacCulloch, R., & Oswald, A. J. (2001). Preferences over inflation and unemployment: Evidence from surveys of happiness. *American Economic Review, 91*(1), 335–341.

Di Tella, R., MacCulloch, R., & Oswald, A. J. (2003). The macroeconomics of happiness. *The Review of Economics and Statistics, 85*(4), 809–827.

Easterlin, R. A. (1974). Does economic growth improve the human lot? Some empirical evidence. In P. David & M. Reder (Eds.), *Nations and households in economic growth: Essays in Honour of Moses Abramovitz*. New York: Academic.

Easterlin, R. A., Morgan, R., Switek, M., & Fei Wang. (2012). China's life satisfaction, 1990–2010. In *Proceedings of the National Academy of Sciences of the United States of America*. http://www.pnas.org/cgi/doi/10.1073/pnas.1205672109. Accessed 27 July 2014.

Folstein, M. F., Folstein, S. E., & McHugh, P. R. (1975). Mini-mental state: A practical method for grading the cognitive state of patients for the clinician. *Journal of Psychiatric Research, 12*, 189–198.

Frey, B. S., & Stutzer, A. (2002, June). What can economists learn from happiness research? *Journal of Economic Literature, 40*(2), 402–435.

[7] We thank one of the anonymous referees on his/her insightful review and constructive suggestions.

Frey, B. S., & Stutzer, A. (2010, September). Happiness and public choice. *Public Choice, 14*, S.557–S.573.

Gao, S., Meng, X., & Zhang, L. (2014). Fiscal decentralization and life satisfaction: Evidence from urban China. *Social Indicators Research, 119*(3), 1177–1194. doi:10.1007/s11205-013-0552-z.

Kahneman, D., & Krueger, A. B. (2006, Winter). Developments in the measurement of subjective well-being. *Journal of Economic Perspectives, 20*(1), 3–24.

Knight, J., & Gunatilaka, R. (2011). Does economic growth raise happiness in China. *Oxford Development Studies, 39*(1), 1–24.

Li, H., & Zhou, L.-A. (2005). Political turnover and economic performance: The incentive role of personnel control in China. *Journal of Public Economics, 89*(9–10), 1743–1762.

Liu, Z., & Shang, Q. (2012). Individual well-being in urban China: The role of income expectations. *China Economic Review, 23*(4), 833–849.

Yamamura, E. (2011). The influence of government size on economic growth and life satisfaction: A case study from Japan. *Japanese Economy, 38*(4), 28–64.

Zeng, Y., Vaupel, J. W., Xiao, Z., Zhang, C., & Liu, Y. (2002). Socio-demographic and health profiles of the oldest old in China. *Population and Development Review, 28*(2), 251–273.

Chapter 8
Leisure Activities and Quality of Life Among Older Adults in Spain

Raul Lardies-Bosque, Gloria Fernandez-Mayoralas, Fermina Rojo-Perez, Maria João Forjaz, Pablo Martinez-Martin, José-Manuel Rojo-Abuin and on behalf of Spanish Research Group on Quality of Life and Ageing

Introduction

Leisure is an important source of personal satisfaction and well-being at all ages, particularly after retirement, when more free time is available (Adams et al. 2011; Fernández-Ballesteros et al. 2001; Kelly et al. 1986; Nimrod 2007; Rowe and Kahn

R. Lardies-Bosque
Department of Geography, Environmental Sciences Institute,
University of Zaragoza, C/ Pedro Cerbuna 12, 50009 Zaragoza, Spain
e-mail: rlardies@unizar.es

G. Fernandez-Mayoralas (✉) • F. Rojo-Perez
Institute of Economics, Geography and Demography (IEGD), Centre for Human and Social Sciences (CCHS), Spanish National Research Council (CSIC),
C/ Albasanz 26-28, 28037 Madrid, Spain
e-mail: gloria.fernandezmayoralas@cchs.csic.es; fermina.rojo@cchs.csic.es

M.J. Forjaz
National School of Public Health and Consortium for Biomedical Research in Neurodegenerative Diseases (CIBERNED), Carlos III Institute of Health, C/ Sinesio Delgado 6, 28029 Madrid, Spain
e-mail: jforjaz@isciii.es

P. Martinez-Martin
National Center of Epidemiology and Consortium for Biomedical Research in Neurodegenerative Diseases (CIBERNED), Carlos III Institute of Health,
Avdª. Monforte de Lemos, 5, 28029 Madrid, Spain
e-mail: pmartinez@isciii.es

J.-M. Rojo-Abuin
Statistical Analysis Unit (UAE) Centre for Human and Social Sciences (CCHS),
Spanish National Research Council (CSIC), C/ Albasanz 26-28, 28037 Madrid, Spain
e-mail: josemanuel.rojo@cchs.csic.es

F. Maggino (ed.), *A New Research Agenda for Improvements in Quality of Life*,
Social Indicators Research Series 57, DOI 10.1007/978-3-319-15904-1_8

1997). What's more, and for several decades now, the importance has become apparent of the positive relationship between elderly people participating in various activities and successful ageing (Havighurst and Albrecht 1953). It has also been established that performing activities helps extend the personal autonomy stage and delay the negative effects of ageing and dependence (IMSERSO 2008; Janke et al. 2008).

The effect of carrying out activities on life satisfaction, as an indicator of overall quality of life (QoL), health and social integration (Agahi et al. 2006; Beckett et al. 2002; Havighurst et al. 1968; Lemon et al. 1972; Wahrendorf and Siegrist 2010) is covered in the theory on carrying out activities at all ages (Havighurst 1961), and also during old age, as adapting to ageing is promoted by high levels of involvement in social and leisure activities and a change of roles when these activities should be abandoned (Adams et al. 2011).

Leisure and social participation activities are also a fundamental cornerstone of active ageing, as conceptualized by the World Health Organization as "the process of optimizing opportunities for health, participation and security in order to enhance quality of life as people age" (World Health Organization 2002). So the possible overlap of meanings between active ageing and quality of life would be confined to a dynamic process in the first case or dynamic state in the second (Bowling 2004).

Despite the evidence of the benefits of social participation and involvement in leisure activities, there has been relatively little research on older adults (Bowling and Stafford 2007), and very little research on type of leisure in old age and factors that explain its carrying out.

For this reason, the goals of this research are to: (i) define the use of free time profiles according to the type of leisure activity performed by older adults in Spain, (ii) analyze the differences in the leisure profile of older adults based on sociodemographic and residential characteristics, and the objective conditions in the most important domains for their QoL, and (iii) obtain an explanatory model of the type/profile of leisure activity to which older adults in Spain belong, knowing their characteristics and objective living conditions.

In accordance with other lines of work (Liang et al. 2013), the basic assumption is that sociodemographic characteristics (such as age, gender, marital status, social class, education, income or occupation, and others of a family nature) are closely related to the QoL of older adults (Han 1988; Pinquart 2001) and are predictors of leisure activity and satisfaction patterns (Agate et al. 2009; Fernández-Ballesteros et al. 2001; Spiers and Walker 2009).

Leisure and Quality of Life of the Elderly: Concepts, Measurement and Research

To tackle the proposed objectives, some methodological and conceptual aspects need to be clarified. The first is the nature and content of leisure, so it is firstly necessary to define what it is, what activities it includes and how they are classified. In scientific literature, leisure is normally related to spare time after performing mandatory activities (Gerstl 1983). In this respect, leisure activities among older adults would be those that do not include work activities, looking after family members or other persons, household chores or educational tasks.

Leisure is classified in various ways (Nimrod 2007), normally grouping activities into two or three types depending on whether they are outdoor or indoor (Neal et al. 1999); active or passive, physical, cognitive or cultural (Näsi et al. 2012), performed individually or collectively (Kleiber 1999), whether they are focused on persons or places (Lloyd and Auld 2002), or are social, creative, artistic, intellectual or sporting in nature (Scott and Willits 1998).

Another methodological consideration is the criteria used to measure leisure activities. One approach is to use objective criteria based on the frequency and time devoted to carrying out various activities (Allen 1991), access to leisure facilities or the frequency of using such facilities (Moller 1992).

While there is no single conceptualization of QoL, and perhaps several scientific reviews, contributions and discussions on this matter (Bowling et al. 2002; Bowling 2004; Brown et al. 2004), it is generally agreed that it is a multidimensional concept. In this respect, it has been confirmed in Spain that after health, family, economic resources and the social network, leisure is the fifth most nominated dimension by the elderly population for expressing understanding of their QoL (Fernández-Mayoralas et al. 2007, 2011), and the interrelationship of these domains largely defines overall QoL in old age (Rojo-Pérez and Fernández-Mayoralas 2011).

Among the associations observed in the literature between different QoL domains and leisure, health appears as an influencing variable, with activities dropping when people suffer mental problems or physical limitations (Paillard-Borg et al. 2009), but which can also benefit from the activities carried out, affecting the maintenance and improvement of physical, mental and intellectual ability (Culos-Reed et al. 2008; Janke et al. 2008; Jenkins et al. 2002; Schooler and Mulatu 2001), control of dementia (Wang et al. 2002), reduction in morbidity (Malmberg et al. 2005) and the risk of mortality (Glass et al. 1999; Lan et al. 2006).

Family and social networks are also factors related to the type of leisure activity performed as they can favour or determine activities during old age (Beckett et al. 2002). Ateca-Amestoy et al. (2008) argue that family obligations such as care giving responsibility may negatively impact on QoL through less leisure satisfaction due to time constraints. Several investigations into determinants of healthy ageing also demonstrate that being engaged in a productive and social activity is associated with wellbeing and QoL improvement (Li and Ferraro 2005;

Litwin 2001; Luoh and Herzog 2002; Mendes de Leon 2005; Wahrendorf et al. 2006).

The role of economic resources in leisure is not only demonstrated with spending power in terms of availability of money (or its perception), but also in the availability of free time, so those individuals who enjoy both of these "riches" will be more likely to participate in leisure activities (Bittman 1998).

Apart from the most important domains for QoL, the residential environment plays a significant role in leisure activities insofar as the greater or lesser provision of amenities may either facilitate or impede participation in certain types of leisure pursuits (sports or cultural facilities, green areas, etc.), which could indirectly affect the promotion of independence for the autonomy and social participation of elderly people (Fernández-Mayoralas et al. 2004; Rojo-Pérez et al. 2001, 2002, 2007a).

In this context, the effect of carrying out activities on the various dimensions of QoL in old age has been confirmed very positively (Ardahan and Mert 2013), and an improvement in living conditions has been perceived too (Silverstein and Parker 2002). Likewise, people who have comparable levels of activity to younger adults, and who even carry out activities which they were not involved in previously, improve their level of well-being (Hooyman and Kiyak 1996).

Material and Methods

The data comes from a face-to-face survey on QoL conducted in 2008 (CadeViMa-España Survey, 2008). A cross-sectional design was used on a sample of community-dwelling older adults. A nationally representative sample made up of 1,106 adults residing in Spain aged 60 years and over was selected from the total population of this age (9,812,307 individuals according to Official Population Figures of the Municipal Register on December 2007; Instituto Nacional de Estadistica, 2007). The allowable error was ±3.5 % for a confidence level of 95 %. A geodemographically based proportional multistage stratified sampling was employed in order to improve representativeness. The first-stage sampling unit was proportional sampling according to Spain's autonomous communities (14 groups) and town population size (seven groups) to assure that all individuals had an equal probability of being selected; the second-stage sampling unit was quota sampling of gender and age (three groups). We excluded 4.6 % of subjects on suspicion of cognitive impairment (score greater than 4 errors in the Short Portable Mental Status Questionnaire) (Pfeiffer 1975). The final sample resulted in a proportional sample by sex, age and geographic location. More information on this survey can be found in Fernandez-Mayoralas et al. (2012).

Table 8.1 shows the variables selected and their distributions and expected ranges:

(a) *Sociodemographic characteristics*: age (60 years old and over), gender, marital status, educational level, economical activity, household type.

Table 8.1 Description of the sample according to the main dimensions of quality of life in old age

		Four main clusters of older adults according to leisure activities performed			
	M ± SD	Inactive	Physical and social	Passive and cultural	Very active and tourist
(N = 1,106 individuals)	n (%)	48.32 %	23.34 %	22.16 %	6.18 %
Sociodemographic characteristics					
Age (years)	72.07 ± 7.83	73.99b	69.49a	71.23a	69.75a
Gender ($p \leq 0.001$)					
Male	483 (43.67)	216 (44.91)	144 (29.94)	93 (19.33)	28 (5.82)
Female	623 (56.33)	316 (50.97)	113 (18.23)	151 (24.35)	40 (6.45)
Marital Status ($p \leq 0.001$)					
Single	75 (6.78)	39 (52.00)	13 (17.33)	18 (24.00)	5 (6.67)
Married or de facto	645 (58.32)	285 (44.25)	177 (27.48)	138 (21.43)	44 (6.83)
Divorced or separated	38 (3.44)	9 (24.32)	11 (29.73)	13 (35.14)	4 (10.81)
Widowed	345 (31.19)	199 (58.19)	54 (15.79)	74 (21.64)	15 (4.39)
Educational level ($p \leq 0.001$)					
No education or incomplete primary	349 (31.56)	232 (66.86)	46 (13.26)	54 (15.56)	15 (4.32)
Primary school	432 (39.06)	189 (43.75)	116 (26.85)	103 (23.84)	24 (5.56)
High school, vocational training or university	324 (29.29)	111 (34.58)	94 (29.28)	87 (27.10)	29 (9.03)
Economical activity ($p \leq 0.001$)					
Working	93 (8.42)	27 (29.03)	31 (33.33)	24 (25.81)	11 (11.83)
Retired	569 (51.54)	270 (47.70)	143 (25.27)	125 (22.08)	28 (4.95)
Housewives	334 (30.25)	174 (52.10)	58 (17.37)	77 (23.05)	25 (7.49)
Pensioners	108 (9.78)	60 (56.60)	24 (22.64)	18 (16.98)	4 (3.77)
Household ($p = 0.171$)					
Living alone	275 (24.86)	135 (49.45)	52 (19.05)	70 (25.64)	16 (5.86)
Not living alone	831 (75.14)	397 (47.95)	205 (24.76)	174 (21.01)	52 (6.28)

(continued)

Table 8.1 (continued)

	M ± SD	Four main clusters of older adults according to leisure activities performed			
		Inactive	Physical and social	Passive and cultural	Very active and tourist
(N = 1,106 individuals)	n (%)	48.32 %	23.34 %	22.16 %	6.18 %
Residential features					
Town population size ($p \leq 0.001$)					
Rural (≤2,000 inhabitants)	113 (10.22)	65 (57.52)	32 (28.32)	14 (12.39)	2 (1.77)
Intermediate (2,001–10,000 inhabitants)	165 (14.92)	94 (56.97)	41 (24.85)	22 (13.33)	8 (4.85)
Urban (≥10,001 inhabitants)	828 (74.86)	373 (45.32)	184 (22.36)	208 (25.27)	58 (7.05)
Accessibility to community services					
Neighborhood level (shops, bars, transport, church)	0.03 ± 0.73	0.11a	–0.02a,b	–0.06b	–0.13a,b
Municipality level (daycare centres, centres for older, cultural and sport services, green zones)	0 ± 0.58	0.05a,b	–0.05a,c,d	–0.08c	0.14b,d
Primary and specialised health services	–0.03 ± 0.55	–0.02a	–0.04a	–0.06a	0.00a
Health conditions					
EQ-5D-3 level version (descriptive system)					
Mobility (EQ-5D-3L) ($p \leq 0.001$)					
I have no problems in walking about	863 (78.03)	364 (42.37)	235 (27.36)	197 (22.93)	63 (7.33)
I have some problems in walking about	238 (21.52)	165 (69.62)	22 (9.28)	45 (18.99)	5 (2.11)
I am confined to bed	5 (0.45)	3 (60.00)	0 (0.00)	2 (40.00)	0 (0.00)
Self-Care (EQ-5D-3L) ($p \leq 0.001$)					
I have no problems with self-care	1,005 (90.87)	450 (44.96)	255 (25.47)	228 (22.78)	68 (6.79)
I have some problems washing or dressing myself	87 (7.87)	70 (81.40)	1 (1.16)	15 (17.44)	0 (0.00)
I am unable to wash or dress myself	14 (1.27)	12 (85.71)	1 (7.14)	1 (7.14)	0 (0.00)
Usual Activities (e.g. work, study, housework, family or leisure activities) (EQ-5D-3L) ($p \leq 0.001$)					
I have no problems with performing my usual activities	911 (82.37)	375 (41.35)	245 (27.01)	219 (24.15)	68 (7.50)

I have some problems with performing my usual activities	178 (16.09)	142 (80.23)	12 (6.78)	23 (12.99)	0 (0.00)
I am unable to perform my usual activities	17 (1.54)	15 (88.24)	0 (0.00)	2 (11.76)	0 (00)
Pain/Discomfort (EQ-5D-3L) ($p \leq 0.001$)					
I have no pain or discomfort	548 (49.55)	217 (39.82)	159 (29.17)	126 (23.12)	43 (7.89)
I have moderate pain or discomfort	475 (42.95)	256 (54.12)	88 (18.60)	105 (22.20)	24 (5.07)
I have extreme pain or discomfort	83 (7.50)	59 (71.08)	10 (12.05)	13 (15.66)	1 (1.20)
Anxiety/Depression (EQ-5D-3 L) ($p \leq 0.001$)					
I am not anxious or depressed	869 (78.57)	379 (43.87)	223 (25.81)	197 (22.8)	65 (7.52)
I am moderately anxious or depressed	202 (18.26)	125 (61.88)	32 (15.84)	42 (20.79)	3 (1.49)
I am extremely anxious or depressed	35 (3.16)	28 (80.00)	2 (5.71)	5 (14.29)	0 (0.00)
EQ-5D-TTO index (−0.65/0.00–1.00)	0.83 ± 0.25	0.76b	0.91a	0.86a	0.94a
EQ-5D-VAS (0–100)	66.22 ± 20.92	59.93b	74.50a	68.77c	74.88a,c
Funtional independence scale (without domestic tasks) (17–51)	49.65 ± 3.87	48.59b	50.84a	50.35a	50.81a
Funtional independence scale (with domestic tasks) (23–69)	64.39 ± 7.59	62.62b	66.10a	65.98a	65.66a
Barthel index (0–100)	95.82 ± 11.05	93.18b	98.76a	97.58a	98.96a
Depression (HADS-D sub scale) (0–21)	4.92 ± 4.29	6.62b	3.22a	3.52a	2.97a
Family and social networks					
Visits/month (family network)	45.39 ± 34.18	45.24a,b	51.61a	41.36b	38.52b,c
Visits/month (best friends and neighbors)	23.55 ± 18.53	22.29b	27.09a	23.45a,b	20.71a,b
Tipology of the household ($p \leq 0.001$)					
Living alone	276 (24.95)	135 (49.27)	53 (19.34)	70 (25.55)	16 (5.84)
Living with a partner	431 (38.97)	175 (40.70)	125 (29.07)	107 (24.88)	23 (5.35)
Living with a partner and others (family and other)	214 (19.35)	110 (51.40)	52 (24.30)	32 (14.95)	20 (9.35)
Living with children and/or grandchildren	69 (6.24)	40 (59.70)	10 (14.93)	12 (17.91)	5 (7.46)
Living with other relatives	116 (10.49)	72 (62.07)	17 (14.66)	23 (19.83)	4 (3.45)

(continued)

Table 8.1 (continued)

		Four main clusters of older adults according to leisure activities performed			
	M ± SD	Inactive	Physical and social	Passive and cultural	Very active and tourist
(N = 1,106 individuals)	n (%)	48.32 %	23.34 %	22.16 %	6.18 %
Economic resources (Income)					
Income (p ≤ 0.001)	813.34 ± 319.26	745.62b	843.27a	876.22a	1010.47c
Less than 300 euros	14 (1.27)	9 (64.29)	2 (14.29)	3 (21.43)	0 (0.00)
301–600 euros	313 (28.30)	197 (63.34)	56 (18.01)	49 (15.76)	9 (2.89)
601–900 euros	418 (37.79)	192 (46.15)	110 (26.44)	98 (23.56)	16 (3.85)
901–1,200 euros	250 (22.60)	97 (38.96)	65 (26.10)	59 (23.69)	28 (11.24)
More than 1,200 euros	111 (10.04)	37 (33.33)	24 (21.62)	35 (31.53)	15 (13.51)
Leisure activities (number)					
Total activities (0–32)	7.84 ± 3.44				
Physical (0–8)	1.96 ± 1.38				
Passive (0–5)	2.90 ± 1.00				
Cultural (0–9)	1.32 ± 1.22				
Social (0–9)	1.60 ± 1.19				
Tourism (0–1)	0.06 ± 0.24				
Quality of life					
Satisfaction with life (0–10)	6.94 ± 1.75	6.61b	7.32a	7.21a	7.24a
PWI (0–100)	71.03 ± 13.50	66.80b	76.12a	73.56a	76.33a

Discriminant analysis showed that 81.9 % of the people were correctly classified in the four clusters
Test of significance for categorical variables: Chi-Square Test
Tests for continuous variables are adjusted for all pair-wise comparisons within a row of each innermost sub-table using the Bonferroni correction
Letters a,b,c,d identify values means with significant differences

(b) *Residential features*: selected here were the size of municipality of residence and three accessibility factors to community services, at a neighbourhood, municipal and primary care and specialist health service level (day centres, senior citizens centres. . .), obtained by a factor analysis of the 11 variables that indicate access time to amenities or services (cultural and sports facilities, green areas. . .), with a total explained variance of 79 % (Rojo-Pérez et al. 2010).

(c) *Health conditions*: The descriptive instrument of health-related QoL and health status EQ-5D-3 level version was used, including the five Dimensions descriptive system (mobility, self-care, usual activities, pain/discomfort, and anxiety/depression), the single index obtained by the trade-off method (EQ-5D-TTO), with a theoretical possible range of −1.00 to 1.00 (Badia et al. 1999), and the visual analogue scale (EQ-5D-VAS), from 0, worst imaginable health state, to 100, best imaginable health state. Concerning functional ability, two scales were included: (1) the Barthel Index (Mahoney and Barthel 1965), a 10-item measure of functional ability of the person in the performance of activities in daily living. The total score ranges from 0 (completely dependent) to 100 (completely independent); and (2) the Functional Independence Scale (FIS), which was specifically created to assess the degree of functional independence in the non-institutionalized older population (Martínez-Martín et al. 2009), considering or not domestic tasks. FIS measures functional independence in several activities of daily living. Each activity has the following response categories: can do it without help, needs help to do it, and cannot do it and someone does it for you. An additional response category – has never done it – is considered for the activities of household duties. This scale was designed and validated for community-dwelling older adults in Spain. Higher scores indicate greater functional independence. Finally, for measuring depression, the depression subscale of the Hospital Anxiety and Depression Scale (HADS-D) was used. HADS-D is a brief self report measure developed to screen depression states in non-psychiatric patients (Zigmond and Snaith 1983). It consists of seven items referring to the past week, rated on a 0–3 Likert-type scale. Scores of 7 or less are considered non-cases; 8–10 are doubtful cases; and 11 or higher indicate depression states.

(d) *Family and Social networks:* apart from typology of household, two variables were used related to contact with the family network and social network (friends and neighbours). From the seven original variables on frequency of contacts (every or almost every day, 1–2 times a week, 1–2 times a month, with less frequency), with different family members (daughters, sons, daughters-in-law/sons-in-law, grandsons/granddaughters, siblings/brothers and sisters in-law, parents/parents-in-law and other relatives), an added variable of monthly contacts was obtained, transferring the original frequency to days/months, with the family network. Following the same procedure, the two original variables on contact with best friends and neighbours resulted in a single variable on monthly contacts with the social network.

(e) *Economic resources*: monthly income in five response categories. Missing values (30.1 %) were estimated through a general linear model, using the number of goods or services that could be afforded (Fernandez-Mayoralas et al. 2012).

(f) *Leisure activities (and free time)*: from the 32 variables on activities questioned in the survey, five variables were obtained by counting the number of activities performed, according to the type of activity and a frequency of at least 1–2 times/month. These variables are the grouped original categories in the questionnaire:

1. Physical activities (eight activities): sport, dancing, looking after a garden or vegetable garden, nature walks, city walks, hunting/fishing, carrying out repairs or DIY at home, going shopping (not to the market).
2. Passive activities (five activities): watching TV/videos, listening to the radio, listening to music, playing cards/board games, doing handicrafts/sewing.
3. Cultural activities (nine activities): going to the cinema, going to the theatre, going to museums/exhibitions, reading newspapers/magazines, reading books, studying/learning new things, playing a musical instrument, painting/drawing, browsing the Internet.
4. Social and participatory activities (nine activities): going to church, voluntary work, involvement in clubs/associations, attending strikes/demonstrations, getting together with friends and neighbours, going to parties, going to sports events, going to restaurants, going to the bingo.
5. Travel and tourism.

(g) *Quality of Life:* two variables were used, one on general life satisfaction, as a single item on an 11 point Likert scale from 0 (completely dissatisfied) to 10 (completely satisfied), and another on subjective well-being; the Personal Wellbeing Index (PWI) (International Wellbeing Group 2006) was obtained from seven domains (standard of living, health, achievement, personal relationships, sense of security, belonging to the community, future security) (Cummins et al. 2003; Rodriguez-Blazquez et al. 2011).

The five variables by counting of the number of leisure activities, with a different range, were standardized to normalize the units of measurement, whereby their mean was 0 and their variance 1. After that, a cluster analysis was carried out to identify homogeneous groups of individuals defined by similar patterns of performing activities (centers/centroids over the standardized mean, 0, in Table 8.2). This classification of people, validated by discriminant analysis, was related by bivariate analysis with selected variables (Table 8.1). Cluster Analysis was run under the non-hierarchical clustering procedure K-means, using the Euclidian distance based on standardized values.

Finally, a Multinomial Logistic Regression Analysis was conducted for each group of variables (sociodemographics, residential, health conditions and functional capacity, family and social networks, and economic resources), taking

Table 8.2 Classification of people according to the leisure activities performed

Number of activities in each category carried out at least 1–2 times a month (standardised)	Conglomerate: final cluster centers/centroids				
	Physical and social	Inactive	Passive and cultural	Very active	Tourists
Physical leisure activities	1.11236	−0.59717	−0.08765	1.16888	0.23215
Passive leisure activities	0.08841	−0.46368	0.81298	0.84755	−0.17188
Cultural leisure activities	0.09516	−0.56929	0.85400	1.71164	0.13049
Social leisure activities	0.67106	−0.65131	0.46171	1.26077	0.42122
Travel, sightseeing	−0.25645	−0.25645	−0.25645	3.89582	3.89582
Total cases (n = 1,101)	257	532	244	39	29
% cases	23.4	48.3	22.2	3.5	2.6

Discriminant analysis shows that 72 % of cases were correctly classified

these as independent variables. The aim was pre-selecting variables that were significant for their inclusion as independent variables in an overall Multinomial Logistic Regression Analysis, where classification of people obtained by cluster analysis was used as dependent variable in order to obtain an explanatory model of the leisure activity profile of older adults in Spain, knowing their characteristics and objective living conditions. For this, the cluster defined and labeled "Inactive people" was used as the reference category (Table 8.3).

The pseudo R^2 Nagelkerke coefficient can be used as a measure of the power of explanation of the model and it was employed in all cases to show the goodness of fit of the models obtained. This coefficient is based on likelihood of the model when the explanation variables are retained (Norusis 2004). Although R^2 Nagelkerke ranges from 0 to 1, values >0.3 can be considered acceptable.

Results

Sample Characteristics

Table 8.1 shows the demographic profile and the living conditions of the population studied (Fernandez-Mayoralas et al. 2012). The sociodemographic and residential profile coincides roughly with the situation that can be seen from the population census data (Rojo-Pérez et al. 2007b).

As for living conditions in the most important dimensions for their QoL, older adults show a relatively good situation with regard to health, functional capacity and Health Related Quality of Life (HRQL), also enjoying a well-connected family and social network. However, their objective conditions with respect to economic resources are unfavourable, as almost two thirds are on an income of less than 900 euros/month.

Table 8.3 Partial and global multinomial logistic regression models: significance coefficients. Dependent variable: classification obtained by cluster analysis and validated by discriminant analysis in four groups of people performing activities over the standardized mean

Variables	Socio – demographics characteristics regression model	Residential features regression model	Health conditions regression model	Family and social networks regression model	Economic resources (income) regression model	Final regression model[a]
Age (years)	0.000					
Gender	0.041					0.000
Marital Status	0.209					
Educational level	0.000					0.000
Economical activity	0.397					
Household	0.295					
Town population size		0.000				0.009
Accessibility to community services						
Neighborhood level (shops, bars, transport, church)		0.005				
Municipality level (daycare centres, centres for older, cultural and sport services, green zones)		0.003				0.005
Primary and specialised health services		0.867				
EQ-5D-TTO index (−0.65/0.00–1.00)			0.126			
EQ-5D-VAS (0–100)			0.000			0.000
Functional independence scale (without domestic tasks) (17–51)			0.034			0.000
Functional independence scale (with domestic tasks) (23–69)			0.056			
Barthel index (0–100)			0.455			

Depression (HADS-D sub scale) (0–21)			0.000			0.000
Visits/month (family network)				0.012		0.011
Visits/month (best friends and neighbors)				0.022		0.017
Tipology of the household				0.000		
Income					0.000	0.000
Pseudo R^2 Nagelkerke	0.154	0.058	0.235	0.062	0.059	0.313

[a]*The model has been controlled by age*

Likewise, this population does not appear to be very active when it comes to leisure and free time, as they barely perform an average of 8 activities of 32 included in the questionnaire and, of these activities, a high average (mean: 3.9; SD: 1.0) are passive in nature (watching TV, listening to the radio, listening to music, playing board games or doing handicrafts such as sewing). Less predominant activities are those of a cultural nature (mean: 1.32; SD: 1.22).

Their overall QoL, measured as general life satisfaction, is high (6.94 ± 1.75), but even more so when considering personal well-being through PWI (71.03 ± 13.50). These results are in line with others obtained in the older adult population in Spain (Rojo-Perez et al. 2012).

Classification of Older Adults According to the Type of Leisure Activity They Perform

The cluster analysis application helped classify people into five basic types of leisure and free time activities (Table 8.2):

Cluster 1: "Physical and social", which accounts for almost a fourth of the population (23.3 %), performing mainly physical activities (sport, dancing, walking…) and, to a lesser extent, social and participatory activities (meeting with family and friends, going to restaurants, participating in NGOs…).

Cluster 2: "Inactive people" was the most numerous group accounting for almost half of interviewees (48.3 % of individuals), who had a low activity profile in carrying out any type of leisure activity; this is indicated by negative values and is therefore below the mean in final cluster centres.

Cluster 3: "Passive and cultural" type made up of just over 22 % of individuals, who devoted their free time to both passive leisure activities (watching TV, listening to the radio, sewing…) and cultural activities (going to the cinema, going to the theatre, studying, browsing the Internet…).

Cluster 4: "Very active people" was a very small group with 3.6 % of interviewees, being people that carry out any type of leisure activity above the mean (positive values of final cluster centres).

Cluster 5: "Tourist people" accounting for only 2.6 % of the population who were notably involved in travel and tourism.

The discriminant analysis shows that these five clusters correctly classify 72 % of the population studied. However, given the small size of types 4 ("Very active") and 5 ("Tourist"), and their similar profile in use of free time in travel and tourism activities, for the subsequent analyses these two groups were considered jointly and the discriminate analysis repeated, obtaining a better and more correct classification (81.9 %). Hence, these 4 homogeneous groups of subjects obtained through Cluster Analysis and validated synthesized the dependent variable used in this paper, using as the reference category the cluster defined and labeled as "Inactive people".

Characteristics of the Population According to Their Activity Profile

Table 8.1 shows the population according to their free time activity profile based on their characteristics and living conditions.

Sociodemographic and Residential Characteristics

The "Inactive" population shows a significantly higher average age (74 years old) than the rest of the groups. There are also differences between them in terms of sex, marital status, educational level and relationship with economic activity, but not in terms of cohabitation (living alone or accompanied by someone).

This group of "Inactive" older adults is dominated by women, singles and widows/widowers, people with pre-primary education levels and housewives and pensioners. However, in the population group with "Physical and social" leisure the opposite categories are more likely: married or divorced men with a primary or higher level of educational studies, still working or retired, while in population groups with "Passive and Cultural" and "Very active and Tourist" leisure there is a notable presence of divorced/separated individuals, people with higher levels of education and still working.

Depending on the size of habitat, "Inactive" population groups with "Physical and Social" leisure predominate in rural or intermediate environments, while "Passive and Cultural" leisure and the "Very active and Tourist" profile is more predominant in urban areas.

Accessibility to neighbourhood and municipal community services is significantly different in the "Inactive" and "Passive and Cultural" groups, being considered greater for the former. Municipal services are also considered more accessible by the population included in the "Very active and Tourist" group than the "Passive and Cultural" group. However, no differences are noticed in accessibility to primary and specialist healthcare services in terms of group or leisure profile.

Health Conditions and Functional Capacity

The EQ-5D descriptive system shows significant differences depending on the leisure and free time activities profile. In the "Inactive" persons group there is a predominance of people with problems in any of the five dimensions (mobility, self-care, usual activities, pain and anxiety/depression). On the other hand, in the "Physical and Social" leisure group, of note is the population category with no problems, pain or anxiety/depression. In this respect, the state of health perceived by the "Inactive" group interviewed is less than 60 % on the EQ-5D-VAS, compared to scores close to 75 % among those involved in "Physical and Social" leisure or in the "Very active and Tourist" group. Therefore, the population grouped in the

"Inactive" cluster is significantly different to the other three groups in the HRQoL EQ-5D-TTO, with barely 0.76 out of 1, compared to scores of above 0.90 among the population in the "Physical and Social" group or from the "Very active and Tourist" group, or above 0.85 among those belonging to the "Passive and Cultural" leisure cluster.

The contrast of means on the Barthel Functional Capacity indices and Functional Independence Scales, and also depression according to the HADS-D, shows that there are significant differences between the "Inactive" population and the rest of the groups, with the latter having proportions close to 100 % free of disability. Consequently, the health conditions and functional capacity of the population in the "Inactive" cluster are significantly different and worse than those observed in the other three groups.

Family and Social Networks

The older adult population that receives the most number of visits a month is classified under the "Physical and Social" leisure profile, with significant differences compared to those in the "Passive and Cultural" and "Very active and Tourist" group in terms of family visits, and the "Inactive" group in terms of visits from friends and neighbours.

People in the "Inactive" group normally live in larger households (with or without a partner but with other people such as sons/daughters, grandsons/granddaughters or other family members); those interviewed in the "Physical and Social" group are mainly married or living with a partner; singles and married couples/people living with a partner predominate in the "Passive and Cultural" leisure profile, while in the "Very active and Tourist" group there is a predominance of those who live with a partner and other people (larger households and with possibly younger members).

Economic Resources

Older adults that make up the "Inactive" cluster, with around 40 % on an income of less than 600 euros/month, have a lower economic level with significant differences compared to the rest of the groups. For its part, the "Very active and Tourist" group, in which 63 % have an income of more than 900 euros/month, has the highest economic level with significant differences compared to the rest of the groups.

Quality of Life and Personal Well-Being

Overall QoL, in terms of general life satisfaction and personal well-being (PWI), is significantly less in the "Inactive" profile population compared to the rest of the groups based on the leisure activities performed. No differences were found among the other three activity profiles.

Factors Explaining the Behaviour or Activity Profile of Older Adults in Spain

Table 8.3 shows the significance coefficients of the variables in the multinomial logistic regression analysis performed. Of the five partial models produced, those with a better goodness of fit are the one that contains the health condition and functional capacity variables and the one that considers the sociodemographic variables, with a pseudo R^2 of 0.235 and 0.154, respectively. Significant among the variables that indicate health conditions and functional capacity were depression, state of health perceived in the EQ-5D-VAS and the average functional capacity with the Functional Independence Scale, without considering the carrying out of domestic activities. Of the sociodemographic variables, only age, sex and educational level showed significant coefficients. The rest of the partial models had a pseudo R^2 close to 0.06, and most of the variables selected were significant, apart from the accessibility factor to primary and specialist health services.

Of the 13 significant variables taken as independent in the overall regression model the following were eliminated: age, the accessibility factor to neighbourhood services and type of household ($p > 0.05$) obtaining a pseudo R^2 of 0.340. A final overall model including only 10 significant variables achieved a pseudo R^2 Nagelkerke of 0.313, which indicates an acceptable relationship between the predictors and the dependent variable and that the model fits well.

The model shows the probability of belonging to an inactive type or profile of activity (Table 8.4). The probability therefore of belonging to the cluster defined as "Physical and Social" leisure, with reference to the "Inactive" cluster, is explained by health conditions and functional capacity i.e., by better health today measured in the EQ-5D-VAS, greater functional independence and less depression or no depression. This activity profile also depends on family and social network conditions in terms of a higher number of visits/month from both family members and friends and neighbours. The beta coefficient in continuous variables is the change (increase or decrease depending of the sign) in log-odds ratio of falling into (in this case) "Physical and Social" leisure category versus the reference category, "Inactive people", resulting from a one-unit increase/decrease in each independent variable, holding the other covariates constant. For its part, a higher educational level would increase the probability of change from an "Inactivity" profile to another characterized by "Physical and Social" leisure in 134.2 % if educational level is improved from pre-primary to primary education studies, and 185.9 % if higher educational studies are attained.

The probability of belonging to the cluster defined by "Passive and Cultural" leisure, with reference to the "Inactive" cluster, is also related to being less

Table 8.4 Final Multinomial Logistic Regression Model on the variable classification of people performing activities over the standardized mean, obtained by cluster analysis and validated by discriminant analysis in four groups[a]

		B	Sig.	Exp (B)
Physical and social[b]	*Constant*	*−16.553*	*0.000*	
	EQ-5D-VAS (0–100)	0.017	0.000	1.018
	Functional independence scale (without domestic tasks) (17–51)	0.283	0.001	1.327
	Depression (HADS-D sub scale) (0–21)	−0.137	0.000	0.872
	Visits/month (family network)	0.005	0.033	1.005
	Visits/month (best friends and neighbors)	0.014	0.003	1.014
	Educational level			
	High school, vocational training or university	1.050	0.000	2.859
	Primary school	0.851	0.000	2.342
	No education or incomplete primary[c]	0	.	.
Passive and cultural[b]	*Constant*	*−4.648*	*0.011*	
	Accessibility fo community services at municipal level (daycare centres, centres for older, cultural and sport services, green zones)	−0.421	0.023	0.656
	Depression (HADS-D sub scale) (0–21)	−0.145	0.000	0.865
	Gender			
	Female	0.452	0.010	1.571
	Male[c]	0	.	.
	Educational level			
	High school, vocational training or university	0.720	0.003	2.055
	Primary school	0.673	0.001	1.961
	No education or incomplete primary[c]	0	.	.
	Town population size			
	Urban ($\geq$10,001 inhabitants)	0.797	0.015	2.220
	Rural ($\leq$2,000 inhabitants)[c]	0	.	.
Very active and tourists[b]	*Constant*	*−17.890*	*0.012*	
	Accessibility to community services at municipal level (daycare centres, centres for older, cultural and sport services, green zones)	0.491	0.023	1.633
	EQ-5D-VAS (0–100)	0.024	0.006	1.024
	Depression (HADS-D sub scale) (0–21)	−0.126	0.013	0.882
	Income	0.002	0.000	1.002

[a]*The model has been controlled by age*
[b]*Cluster reference category is "Inactive"*
[c]*Reference category in the categorical variable*

depressed, as a health condition; to sociodemographic characteristics such as sex (a 57 % higher probability among women than men) and educational level (96.1 % among those who have completed primary education compared to those with pre-primary studies, and 105.5 % with post-primary studies); belonging to the "Passive and Cultural" leisure group is also explained by the characteristics of the area of residence, such as size of habitat (a 122 % higher probability if living in an urban area compared to a rural environment, without significant differences in the intermediate size) or less accessibility (minus symbol) to municipal services and day centres, senior citizens centres, cultural and sports services and green areas.

Finally, the probability of belonging to the cluster defined as "Very active and Tourist" leisure, with reference to "Inactive" older adults, is explained by two health conditions: once again being less depressed and having better health today in the EQ-5D-VAS, as well as by greater accessibility to municipal services and a higher level of income.

Discussion and Conclusions

This work is a continuation of previous research on the interrelationship between performing leisure activities and well-being and quality of life in old age (Adams et al. 2011; Ardahan and Lapa 2010; Becchetti et al. 2012), focusing on the study of leisure and free time activities in a significant sample of the older adult population living in the community in Spain and factors related to the main dimensions of QoL, as a result of active ageing.

The first finding in the analysis was the obtaining of four uniform groups of older adults according to their activity profile, with the predominance of inactive people, hardly any general involvement in any type of leisure activity and the fundamentally passive nature of the activities carried out, which suggests that retirement or retiring from other main activities does not always move in parallel with active ageing in terms of performing leisure and free time activities.

This result is in line with those obtained in other studies which highlight the inverse relationship between ageing and participating in activities, particularly when health conditions worsen (Ardahan and Lapa 2010; Fernández-Mayoralas et al. 2007; Lardiés-Bosque 2011). Pérez Ortiz (2007) also found that the oldest segment of the population in Spain spends the most amount of time each day on sedentary and solitary activities; moreover, according to the *Survey on Cultural Habits and Practices in Spain 2010–2011* (Ministerio de Cultura 2011), it is observed that passive activities predominate among the oldest age group.

Gender differences in the distribution of the type of leisure activity have also been observed in other research (Avramov and Maskova 2003; IMSERSO 2004; Lardiés-Bosque et al. 2013; Paillard-Borg et al. 2009), and are notable in our study, being shown as a variable associated with both the number and type of activities performed. The empirical evidence suggests that being a man is associated with carrying out a higher number of activities, mainly physical and social in nature, while women do fewer activities that are domestic in nature, i.e. mainly passive, although cultural too. In this respect, Western literature has shown that women are generally at a disadvantage when it comes to participating in leisure activities (Henderson 1996; Lardiés-Bosque 2011); regarding quantity of activities, researchers conclude that women are slightly more constrained in their leisure than men, as their time is often limited by the role expected of them socially in the family with household tasks, and caring for children or elderly parents (Rojek 2006). Women continue to shoulder the majority of household responsibilities regardless of employment outside home, and caring behaviour may lead women to prioritize others' leisure before their own (IMSERSO 2008; Ziegler 2012).

Previous research has also confirmed the importance of educational level in performing leisure activities (Heikkinen et al. 1987; Herzog et al. 1998; Lassey and Lassey 2001; Paillard-Borg et al. 2009). The importance of this factor among older adults in Spain on the amount and type of leisure activities has been confirmed, explaining particularly activity profiles defined by "Physical and Social" and "Passive and Cultural" leisure. Higher education not only provides knowledge, but also broadens individual horizons by providing a basis for many different forms of social activities (Haller et al. 2013). In this respect, it is worth remembering that the older adult population in Spain is characterised by having a low educational level (39 % of the sample only has primary education and 31.5 % does not have any education or failed to finish their studies), which is in general inferior to that noted in other European countries (Fagerström et al. 2007).

With regard to this, economic resources, in terms of the income of older adults, is another significant variable, particularly for defining a "Very Active and Tourist" leisure profile, whereby having a higher level of income would promote greater leisure activity in general and going on more trips and doing more sightseeing in particular. These results support the activity theory, which maintains that income either facilitates or limits choice of leisure activities (Bittman 1998). Specifically, first White (1975) and later other authors (Lee et al. 2001; Scott and Munson 1994; Solop et al. 2001) confirmed the association between an increase in income and increasing outdoor recreation participation by affirming that the main determinants are age and income.

However, among the most important dimensions for QoL in old age, health conditions and functional conditions appear to be particularly important factors in explaining the amount and type of leisure performed (Adams et al. 2011; Paillard-Borg et al. 2009). Functional conditions are particularly significant for defining the "Physical and Social" leisure profile which may be limited by restricted functional capacity (Clark 1996; Schooler and Mulatu 2001). Also, perceived health, as a general indicator of health conditions, would explain belonging to activity profiles based on "Physical and Social" and "Very active and Tourist" leisure (Jenkins et al. 2002). And depression, as a mental health condition, would be a centrally important factor as it would be present in the explanatory models for defining all activity profiles, "Physical and Social", "Passive and Cultural" and "Very active and Tourist", in contrast to the "Inactivity" profile, confirming the close relationship between performing any type of activity and not having depression (Heo et al. 2010; Herzog et al. 1998).

Family and social networks have proved vital for explaining the activity profile based on "Physical and Social" leisure, with people in this group receiving the most number of visits from family members and/or friends. In this context, other authors have discovered a positive relationship between maintaining social ties with family members, friends and neighbours, with greater life satisfaction and well-being in old age (Lemon et al. 1972; Litwin and Shiovitz-Ezra 2006). Specifically, in our study, those who perform "Physical and Social" leisure activities stated that they perceive greater QoL and subjective well-being.

Apart from the above factors, certain contextual residential type variables correlated with the amount and type of leisure activity performed. Bowling and Stafford (2007) found an association between living in urban areas and access to facilities, which would make more active leisure, travelling and tourism and participation in social activities more likely. In our research, living in an urban environment explained an activity profile based on "Passive and Cultural" leisure, while greater accessibility to municipal amenities explained a "Very active and Tourist" leisure profile. However, other aspects did not appear to help define the activity profile based on "Physical and Social" leisure, and other relationships were ambiguous, such as less accessibility to amenities for those belonging to the "Passive and Cultural" leisure group, perhaps because of the predominantly passive nature of the activities, essentially domestic in nature, in characterising this profile. In any case, the role of environmental characteristics when carrying out leisure activities has also been described in other research in Spain (Rojo-Pérez et al. 2007a, b), and Pain et al. (2000) corroborate this by pointing out the importance of the place of residence and its conditions, given that certain age-graded spaces lead to the exclusion or marginalisation of older people in society.

In short, among the factors analysed, health conditions as an individual ages appear to affect the performing of certain types of leisure activities, such that perceiving good health, not having depression or pain and enjoying mobility would explain a very active, physical, social and cultural leisure profile. Certain sociodemographic variables and factors related to the family, social and residential environment were also a very important part of the explanation, particularly of social leisure, in contrast to other aspects such as marital status or certain types of cohabitation which were not related to any activity profile. For their part, economic resources had a central part to play in defining greater activity and particularly travel and tourism-based leisure.

This is the context for the association obtained between number and type of leisure activities with life satisfaction and subjective well-being. In line with other studies, satisfaction and well-being were higher among older adults with a high activity profile based mainly on physical and social leisure (Li and Ferraro 2005; Litwin 2001; Luoh and Herzog 2002; Mendes de Leon 2005; Wahrendorf et al. 2006), while those who reported a lower level of activity also showed lower subjective well-being and life satisfaction. In this respect, life satisfaction has been found to be negatively correlated with passive activities as TV viewing (Frey et al. 2007) by reducing, indirectly, of the time spent in relational activities (Bruni and Stanca 2008). However, in our research, an activity profile based on passive leisure combined with cultural leisure showed a high level of life satisfaction and subjective well-being in contrast to the inactivity profile.

These results support the theory of the activity (Lemon et al. 1972) and assertion that more leisure activities would improve living conditions (Hooyman and Kiyak 1996; Silverstein and Parker 2002), increasing subjective well-being and QoL (Ardahan and Mert 2013).

However, these results are explained in a cultural context and for a population group that has had specific living conditions. Many older adults have lived a life of survival in which the daily grind has restricted them to just trying to survive (Del Barrio 2007), which would explain their limited ability to use their time for leisure activities. It is therefore expected that activities carried out by this age group will change in the future, bearing in mind factors such as greater education and training and increased life expectancy. Consequently, and because the characteristics of the elderly population will also change, the importance of one set of factors or another in the future will vary too.

This work, as with others attempting to explain in other nations participation in leisure and associated well-being (Fagerström et al. 2007; Liang et al. 2013), may lose its validity because of the difficulty of its generalisation due to the lack of intercultural leisure theories and methodological developments in comparative international studies. Despite demonstrating many associations, cross-cultural comparative studies on QoL have been mainly confined to industrialized countries in European and American nations, still being scarce in other cultures (Diener and Suh 1998). Indeed, in Europe, whether or not subjective data on older people's QoL is particularly opposite in a comparative European context where expectations may differ markedly due to the substantial variations in standards of living between older people in different countries (Polverini and Lamura 2005; Weidekamp-Maicher and Reichert 2005). For this reason, discovering internationally and comparatively the different factors that affect the QoL of the elderly remains a challenge for future research (Fagerström et al. 2007).

Acknowledgements This study was supported by the Ministry of Science and Innovation R + D + i National Plan, Refs.: SEJ 2006-15122-C02-01 and SEJ 2006-15122-C02-02.

The following members of the Spanish Research Group on Quality of Life and Ageing are also acknowledged: Gloria Fernández-Mayoralas, Fermina Rojo-Pérez and Karim Ahmed-Mohamed at the Spanish National Research Council (CSIC); M. João Forjaz, Carmen Rodríguez-Blázquez and Alba Ayala at the Institute of Health Carlos III; Pablo Martínez-Martín, Belén Frades-Payo, Beatriz León-Salas and Marina Ávila at the Research Unit, CIEN Foundation, Institute of Health Carlos III, Alzheimer Center Reina Sofia Foundation; Raúl Lardiés-Bosque at the University of Zaragoza; María Eugenia Prieto-Flores at UNED-Open University; and Salomé Martín-García and Iluminada Martínez-López at EULEN Socio-sanitary services.

References

Adams, K. B., Leibbrandt, S., & Moon, H. (2011). A critical review of the literature on social and leisure activity and wellbeing in later life. *Ageing and Society, 31*(4), 683–712.

Agahi, N., Ahacic, K., & Parker, M. G. (2006). Continuity of leisure participation from middle age to old age. *The Journals of Gerontology Series B: Psychological Sciences and Social Sciences, 61*(6), S340–S346.

Agate, J. R., Zabriskie, R. B., Agate, S. T., & Poff, R. (2009). Family leisure satisfaction and satisfaction with family life. *Journal of Leisure Research, 41*(2), 205–223.

Allen, L. (1991). Benefits of leisure services to community satisfaction. In B. L. Driver, P. J. Brown, & G. L. Peterson (Eds.), *Benefits of leisure* (pp. 332–350). State College: Venture Publishing Inc.

Ardahan, F., & Lapa, T. (2010). Outdoor recreation: The reasons and carried benefits for attending outdoor sports of the participants of cycling and/or trekking activities. *International Journal of Human Sciences, 8*(1), 1327–1341.

Ardahan, F., & Mert, M. (2013). Impacts of outdoor activities, demographic variables and emotional intelligence on life satisfaction: An econometric application of a case in Turkey. *Social Indicators Research, 113*(3), 887–901.

Ateca-Amestoy, V., Serrano-del-Rosal, R., & Vera-Toscano, E. (2008). The leisure experience. *Journal of Socio-Economics, 37*(1), 64–78.

Avramov, D., & Maskova, M. (2003). *Active ageing in Europe* (Population series, 1, p. 41). Strasbourg: Council of Europe.

Badia, X., Montserrat, S., Roset, M., & Herdman, M. (1999). Feasibility, validity and test-retest reliability of scaling methods for health states: The visual analogue scale and the time trade-off. *Quality of Life Research, 8*(4), 303–310.

Becchetti, L., Giachin Ricca, E., & Pelloni, A. (2012). The relationship between social leisure and life satisfaction: Causality and policy implications. *Social Indicators Research, 108*(3), 453–490.

Beckett, M., Goldman, N., Weinstein, M., Lin, I.-F., & Chuang, Y.-L. (2002). Social environment, life challenge, and health among the elderly in Taiwan. *Social Science and Medicine, 55*(2), 191–209.

Bittman, M. (1998, November 25–27). Social participation and family welfare: The money and time costs of leisure. In *Changing families, challenging futures*. 6th Australian Institute of Family Studies Conference, Melbourne. http://www.aifs.gov.au/conferences/aifs6/bittman.html. Accessed 8 Nov 2012.

Bowling, A. (2004). A taxonomy and overview of quality of life. In J. Brown, A. Bowling, & T. Flynn (Eds.), *Models of quality of life: A taxonomy and systematic review of the literature*. FORUM Project, European Forum on Population Ageing Research, University of Sheffield, Sheffield.

Bowling, A., & Stafford, M. (2007). How do objective and subjective assessments of neighbourhood influence social and physical functioning in older age? Findings from a British survey of ageing. *Social Science and Medicine, 64*(12), 2533–2549.

Bowling, A., Bannister, D., Sutton, S., et al. (2002). A multidimensional model of the quality of life in older age. *Ageing and Mental Health, 6*(4), 355–371.

Brown, J., Bowling, A., & Flynn, T. (2004). *Models of quality of life: A taxonomy and systematic review of the literature*. FORUM Project, European Forum on Population Ageing Research, University of Sheffield, Sheffield. http://www.shef.ac.uk/ageingresearch

Bruni, L., & Stanca, L. (2008). Watching alone: Relational goods, television and happiness. *Journal of Economic Behavior & Organization, 65*(3–4), 506–528.

Clark, D. O. (1996). The effect of walking on lower body disability among older blacks and whites. *American Journal of Public Health, 86*(1), 57–61.

Culos-Reed, S. N., Stephenson, L., Doyle-Baker, P. K., & Dickinson, J. A. (2008). Mall walking as a physical activity option: Results of a pilot project. *Canadian Journal on Aging/La Revue Canadienne du Vieillissement, 27*(1), 81–87.

Cummins, R. A., Eckersley, R., Pallant, J., Van Vugt, J., & Misajon, R. (2003). Developing a national index of subjective wellbeing: The Australian unity wellbeing index. *Social Indicators Research, 64*(2), 159–190.

Del Barrio, E. (2007). Uso del tiempo entre las personas mayores. *Boletín sobre el Envejecimiento; perfiles y tendencias*, 27 (45pp.). Observatorio de Personas Mayores, Portal Mayores. Madrid: Ministerio de Trabajo y Asuntos Sociales, Secretaría de Estado de Servicios Sociales.

Diener, E., & Suh, E. M. (1998). Age and subjective well-being: An international analysis. *Annual Review of Gerontology and Geriatrics, 17*, 304–324.
Fagerström, C., Borg, C., Balducci, C., Burholt, V., Wenger, C. G., Ferring, D., Weber, G., Holst, G., & Hallberg, I. R. (2007). Life satisfaction and associated factors among people aged 60 years and above in six European countries. *Applied Research in Quality of Life, 2*(1), 33–50.
Fernandez-Ballesteros, R., Zamarron, M. D., & Ruiz, A. (2001). The contribution of socio-demographic and psychosocial factors to life satisfaction. *Ageing and Society, 21*(1), 25–43.
Fernández-Mayoralas, G., Rojo-Pérez, F., & Rojo-Abuín, J. M. (2004). Components of the residential environment and socio-demographic characteristics of the elderly. *Journal of Housing for the Elderly, 18*(1), 25–49.
Fernández-Mayoralas, G., Rojo-Pérez, F., Prieto-Flores, M. E., León-Flores, B., Martínez-Martín, P., Forjaz, M. J., Frades-Payo, B., & García, C. (2007). El significado de la salud en la calidad de vida de los mayores. *Portal Mayores, Informes Portal Mayores, 74*, Madrid. http://envejecimiento.csic.es/documentacion/biblioteca/registro.htm?id=52203. Accessed 25 May 2013.
Fernández-Mayoralas, G., Rojo-Pérez, F., Frades-Payo, B., Martínez-Martín, P., & Forjaz, M. J. (2011). La calidad de vida de los mayores nominada y evaluada por ellos mismos a partir del instrumento SEIQoL-DW. In F. Rojo-Pérez & G. Fernández-Mayoralas (Eds.), *Calidad de vida y envejecimiento: la visión de los mayores sobre sus condiciones de vida* [Quality of later life: The old people perception on their living conditions] (pp. 83–112). Madrid: Fundación BBVA.
Fernandez-Mayoralas, G., Giraldez-Garcia, C., Forjaz, M. M., Rojo-Perez, F., Martinez-Martin, P., & Prieto-Flores, M. E. (2012). Design, measures and sample characteristics of the CadeViMa-Spain survey on quality of life in community-dwelling older adults. *International Psychogeriatrics, 24*(3), 425–438.
Frey, B. S., Benesch, C., & Stutzer, A. (2007). Does watching TV make us happy? *Journal of Economic Psychology, 28*(3), 283–313.
Gerstl, J. (1983). The fine art of leisure. *Management World, 12*, 8–10.
Glass, T., Mendes de León, C., Marottoli, R. A., & Berkman, L. F. (1999). Population based study of social productive activities as predictors of survival among elderly Americans. *British Medical Journal, 319*(7208), 478–483.
Haller, M., Hadler, M., & Kaup, G. (2013). Leisure time in modern societies: A new source of boredom and stress? *Social Indicators Research, 111*(2), 403–434.
Han, S. (1988). The relationship between life satisfaction and flow in elderly Korean immigrants. In M. Csikszentmihalyi & I. S. Csikszentmihalyi (Eds.), *Optimal experience: Psychological studies of flow in consciousness* (pp. 138–149). New York: Cambridge University Press.
Havighurst, R. J. (1961). Successful aging. *The Gerontologist, 1*(1), 8–13.
Havighurst, R. J., & Albrecht, R. (1953). *Older people*. New York: Longman, Green and Company.
Havighurst, R. J., Neugarten, B. L., & Tobin, S. S. (1968). Disengagement and patterns of aging. In B. L. Neugarten (Ed.), *Middle age and aging: A reader in social psychology* (pp. 161–172). Chicago: University of Chicago Press.
Heikkinen, E., Karhu, I., & Jokela, J. (1987). Physical exercise and related factors among elderly people in four European localities. In S. Harris, E. Heikkinen, & W. S. Harris (Eds.), *Physical activity, aging and sports* (Vol. 1, pp. 157–177). Albany: Center for the Study of Aging.
Henderson, K. A. (1996). One size doesn't fit all: The meanings of women's leisure. *Journal of Leisure Research, 28*(3), 139–154.
Heo, J., Lee, Y., McCormick, B. P., & Pedersen, P. M. (2010). Daily experience of serious leisure, flow and subjective well-being of older adults. *Leisure Studies, 29*(2), 207–225.
Herzog, A. R., Markus, H. R., Franks, M. M., & Holmberg, D. (1998). Activities and well-being in older age: Effects of self-concept and educational attainment. *Psychology and Aging, 13*(2), 179–185.
Hooyman, N., & Kiyak, H. A. (1996). *Social gerontology: A multidisciplinary perspective* (4th ed.). Boston: Allyn & Bacon.

IMSERSO. (2004). *Encuesta de condiciones de vida de los mayores, study 4,*597. Madrid: Instituto de Mayores y Servicios Sociales. http://envejecimiento.csic.es/estadisticas/encuestas/index.html. Accessed 12 Apr 2013.

IMSERSO. (2008). *La participación social de las Personas Mayores*. Collection Estudios, Serie Personas Mayores, 11,005. Madrid: Secretaría de Estado de Política Social, Familias y Atención a la Dependencia y a la Discapacidad, Instituto de Mayores y Servicios Sociales (IMSERSO), Ministerio de Educación, Política Social y Deporte.

International Wellbeing Group. (2006). *Personal wellbeing index* (4th ed.). Melbourne: Australian Centre on Quality of Life, Deakin University.

Janke, M. C., Payne, L. L., & Puymbroeck, M. V. (2008). The role of informal and formal leisure activities in the disablement process. *The International Journal of Aging and Human Development, 67*(3), 231–257.

Jenkins, K. R., Pienta, A. M., & Horgas, A. L. (2002). Activity and health-related quality of life in continuing care retirement communities. *Research on Aging, 24*(1), 124–149.

Kelly, J. R., Steinkamp, M., & Kelly, J. R. (1986). Later life leisure: How they play in Peoria. *The Gerontologist, 26*(5), 531–537.

Kleiber, D. A. (1999). *Leisure experience and human development*. New York: Basic Books.

Lan, T.-Y., Chang, H.-Y., & Tai, T.-Y. (2006). Relationship between components of leisure physical activity and mortality in Taiwanese older adults. *Preventive Medicine, 43*(1), 36–41.

Lardiés-Bosque, R. (2011). Ocio, tiempo libre y calidad de vida en la población mayor. In F. Rojo-Pérez & G. Fernández-Mayoralas (Eds.), *Calidad de vida y envejecimiento: la visión de los mayores sobre sus condiciones de vida* (pp. 235–270). Bilbao: Fundación BBVA.

Lardiés-Bosque, R., Rojo-Pérez, F., Rodríguez-Rodríguez, V., Fernández-Mayoralas, G., Prieto Flores, M. E., Ahmed-Mohamed, K., & Rojo-Abuín, J. M. (2013). Actividades de ocio y calidad de vida de los mayores en la Comunidad de Madrid. *Boletín de la Asociación de Geógrafos Españoles, 63*, 493–497.

Lassey, W. R., & Lassey, M. L. (2001). *Quality of life for older people. An international perspective*. Upper Saddle River: Prentice Hall.

Lee, J., Scott, D., & Floyd, M. F. (2001). Structural inequalities in outdoor recreation participation: A multiple hierarchy stratification perspective. *Journal of Leisure Research, 33*(4), 427–449.

Lemon, B. W., Bengtson, V. L., & Peterson, J. A. (1972). An exploration of the activity theory of aging: Activity types and life satisfaction among in-movers to a retirement community. *Journal of Gerontology, 27*(4), 511–523.

Li, Y., & Ferraro, K. F. (2005). Volunteering and depression in later life: Social benefit or selection process? *Journal of Health and Social Behavior, 46*(1), 68–84.

Liang, J., Yamashita, T., & Brown, J. S. (2013). Leisure satisfaction and quality of life in China, Japan, and South Korea: A comparative study using AsiaBarometer 2006. *Journal of Happiness Studies, 14*(3), 753–769.

Litwin, H. (2001). Activity, social network and well-being in old age: An empirical examination. *The Canadian Journal on Aging/La Revue Canadienne du Vieillissement, 19*(3), 343–362.

Litwin, H., & Shiovitz-Ezra, S. (2006). The association between activity and wellbeing in later life: What really matters? *Ageing and Society, 26*(2), 225–242.

Lloyd, K. M., & Auld, C. J. (2002). The role of leisure in determining quality of life: Issues of content and measurement. *Social Indicators Research, 57*(1), 43–71.

Luoh, M. C., & Herzog, A. R. (2002). Individual consequences of volunteer and paid work in old age: Health and mortality. *Journal of Health and Social Behavior, 43*(4), 490–509.

Mahoney, F. I., & Barthel, D. W. (1965). Functional evaluation: The Barthel index. *Maryland State Medical Journal, 14*, 61–65.

Malmberg, J., Miilunpalo, S., Pasanen, M., Vuori, I., & Oja, P. (2005). Characteristics of leisure time physical activity associated with risk of decline in perceived health – A 10-year follow-up of middle-aged and elderly men and women. *Preventive Medicine, 41*(1), 141–150.

Martínez-Martín, P., Fernández-Mayoralas, G., Frades Payo, B., Rojo-Pérez, F., Petidier, R., Rodríguez-Rodríguez, V., Forjaz, M. J., Prieto Flores, M. E., & de Pedro Cuesta, J. (2009). Validation of the functional independence scale. *Gaceta Sanitaria, 23*(1), 49–54.

Mendes de Leon, C. F. (2005). Social engagement and successful aging. *European Journal of Ageing, 2*(1), 64–66.
Ministerio de Cultura. (2011). *Encuesta de Hábitos y Prácticas Culturales en España 2010–2011* (Síntesis de resultados). Madrid: Ministerio de Cultura.
Moller, V. (1992). Spare time use and perceived well-being among black South African youth. *Social Indicators Research, 26*(4), 309–351.
Näsi, M., Räsänen, P., & Sarpila, O. (2012). ICT activity in later life: Internet use and leisure activities amongst senior citizens in Finland. *European Journal of Ageing, 9*(2), 169–176.
Neal, J. D., Sirgy, M. J., & Uysal, M. (1999). The role of satisfaction with leisure travel/tourism services en experiences in satisfaction with leisure life and overall life. *Journal of Business Research, 44*(3), 153–163.
Nimrod, G. (2007). Retirees' leisure: Activities, benefits, and their contribution to life satisfaction. *Leisure Studies, 26*(1), 65–80.
Norusis, M. J. (2004). *SPSS 13.0: Advanced statistical procedures companion*. Upper Saddle River: Prentice Hall.
Paillard-Borg, S., Wang, H.-X., Winblad, B., & Fratiglioni, L. (2009). Pattern of participation in leisure activities among older people in relation to their health conditions and contextual factors: A survey in a Swedish urban area. *Ageing and Society, 29*(5), 803–821.
Pain, R., Mowl, G., & Talbot, C. (2000). Difference and the negotiation of 'old age'. *Environment and Planning D: Society and Space, 18*(3), 377–393.
Pérez Ortiz, L. (2007). Actividades, actitudes y valores, Chap. 6. In *Las personas mayores en España. Informe 2006* (Datos estadísticos estatales, Vol. 1). Madrid: IMSERSO.
Pfeiffer, E. (1975). A short portable mental status questionnaire for the assessment of organic brain deficit in elderly patients. *Journal of the American Geriatric Society, 23*(10), 433–441.
Pinquart, M. (2001). Age differences in perceived positive affect, negative affect, and affect balance in middle and old age. *Journal of Happiness Studies, 2*(4), 375–405.
Polverini, F., & Lamura, G. (2005). Italy: Quality of life in old age I. In A. Walker (Ed.), *Growing older in Europe* (pp. 55–82). Maidenhead: Open University Press.
Rodriguez-Blazquez, C., Frades-Payo, B., Forjaz, M. J., Ayala, A., Martinez-Martin, P., Fernandez-Mayoralas, G., & Rojo-Perez, F., on behalf of the Spanish Group on Quality of Life and Ageing. (2011). Psychometric properties of the International Wellbeing Index in community-dwelling older adults. *International Psychogeriatrics, 23*(1), 161–169.
Rojek, C. (2006). The structural characteristics of modern leisure practice. In C. Rojek, S. M. Shaw, & A. Veal (Eds.), *Handbook of leisure studies* (pp. 13–33). Hampshire: Palgrave.
Rojo-Pérez, F., & Fernández-Mayoralas, G. (2011). Los determinantes subjetivos en la calidad de vida en la vejez y factores explicativos. In F. Rojo (Ed.), *Calidad de Vida y Envejecimiento: la visión de los mayores sobre sus condiciones de vida* (pp. 339–360). Madrid/Bilbao: Fundación BBVA.
Rojo-Pérez, F., Fernández-Mayoralas, G., Pozo-Rivera, E., & Rojo-Abuín, J. M. (2001). Ageing in place: Predictors of the residential satisfaction of elderly. *Social Indicators Research, 54*(2), 173–208.
Rojo-Pérez, F., Fernández-Mayoralas, G., Pozo-Rivera, E., & Rojo-Abuín, J. M. (2002). *Envejecer en casa: la satisfacción residencial de los mayores en Madrid como indicador de su calidad de vida* (Col. Monografías, 23). Madrid: Consejo Superior de Investigaciones Científicas.
Rojo-Pérez, F., Fernández-Mayoralas, G., Rodríguez-Rodríguez, V., Prieto-Flores, M. E., & Rojo-Abuín, J. M. (2007a). Entorno residencial de los mayores en España. Hacia una clasificación municipal. *Boletín de la Asociación de Geógrafos Españoles, 43*, 51–72.
Rojo-Pérez, F., Fernández-Mayoralas, G., Rodríguez-Rodríguez, V., & Rojo-Abuín, J. M. (2007b). The environments of ageing in the context of the global quality of life among the elderly living in family housing. In H. Mollenkopf & A. Walker (Eds.), *Quality of life in old age. International and multi-disciplinary perspectives* (Social indicators research series, Vol. 31, pp. 123–150). Dordrecht: Springer.

Rojo-Pérez, F., Fernández-Mayoralas, G., Forjaz, M. J., Martínez-Martín, P., Lardiés-Bosque, R., & Rojo-Abuín, J. M. (2010). Autonomía y entorno residencial como factores de calidad de vida en población adulta-mayor. *Revista Española de Geriatría y Gerontología, 45*(esp. congr.), 135.

Rojo-Perez, F., Fernandez-Mayoralas, G., Rodriguez-Rodriguez, V., Forjaz, M. J., Rodriguez-Blazquez, C., Prieto-Flores, M. E., Rojo-Abuin, J. M., & Martinez-Martin, P. (2012). The personal wellbeing among community-dwelling older adults in Spain and associated factors. *Journal of Social Research and Policy, 3*(2), 67–94.

Rowe, J. W., & Kahn, R. L. (1997). Successful aging. *The Gerontologist, 37*(4), 433–440.

Schooler, C., & Mulatu, M. S. (2001). The reciprocal effects of leisure time activities and intellectual functioning in older people: A longitudinal analysis. *Psychology and Aging, 16* (3), 466–482.

Scott, D., & Munson, W. (1994). Perceived constraints to park usage among individuals with low incomes. *Journal of Park and Recreation Administration, 12*(4), 79–96.

Scott, D., & Willits, F. K. (1998). Adolescent and adult leisure patterns: A reassessment. *Journal of Leisure Research, 30*(3), 319–330.

Silverstein, M., & Parker, M. G. (2002). Leisure activities and quality of life among the oldest old in Sweden. *Research on Aging, 24*(5), 528–547.

Solop, F. I., Hagen, K. K., & Ostergen, D. (2001). Back to nature: Visiting or not visiting our national parks. *Public Perspective, 12*(4), 41–43.

Spiers, A., & Walker, G. (2009). The effects of ethnicity and leisure satisfaction on happiness, peacefulness, and quality of life. *Leisure Science, 31*(1), 84–99.

Wahrendorf, M., & Siegrist, J. (2010). Are changes in productive activities of older people associated with changes in their well-being? Results of a longitudinal European study. *European Journal of Ageing, 7*(2), 59–68.

Wahrendorf, M., Knesebeck, O., & Siegrist, J. (2006). Social productivity and well-being of older people: Baseline results from the SHARE study. *European Journal of Ageing, 3*(2), 67–73.

Wang, H.-X., Karp, A., Winblad, B., & Fratiglioni, L. (2002). Late-life engagement in social and leisure activities is associated with a decreased risk of dementia: A longitudinal study from the Kungsholmen project. *American Journal of Epidemiology, 155*(12), 1081–1087.

Weidekamp-Maicher, M., & Reichert, M. (2005). Germany: Quality of life in old age I. In A. Walker (Ed.), *Growing older in Europe* (pp. 33–54). Maidenhead: Open University Press.

White, T. H. (1975). Relative importance of education and income as predictors in outdoor recreation participation. *Journal of Leisure Research, 7*(3), 191–199.

World Health Organization. (2002). *Active ageing: A policy framework*. Geneva: WHO.

Ziegler, F. (2012). "You have to engage with life, or life will go away": An intersectional life course analysis of older women's social participation in a disadvantaged urban area. *Geoforum, 43*(6), 1296–1305.

Zigmond, A. S., & Snaith, R. P. (1983). The hospital anxiety and depression scale. *Acta Psychiatrica Scandinavica, 67*(6), 361–370.

Chapter 9
Subjective Well-Being After the Onset of the Need for Personal Assistance and Care

Stefan Weick

Introduction

With the rise of life expectancy, the number of elderly individuals in need of personal assistance is growing. Most of the care is provided by private households. The help of family members, partly supported by nursing services, allows many of those in need of personal assistance and nursing care to remain in their usual living environment. Nonetheless, one can assume that this has serious effects on the quality of life of those affected, who are dependent in varying degrees on the help of others. Reliance on the help of other people is associated with many restrictions in everyday life, and thus affects subjective well-being in different areas of life. This paper first gives an overview of the risk of requiring assistance over the life course, and of the situation of the individuals affected. The paper focuses on changes in life satisfaction in relation to the academic discussion on the processes of adaptation to changing circumstances. In recent years, 'set point theory' has taken on a central role in explaining subjective well-being, but revisions of the theory have been called for (Diener et al. 2006; Headey 2006; Lucas et al. 2003). The starting points for this theory are aspiration adaptation theory and the assumptions of personality psychology. According to these, people have a stable satisfaction level that is based on genetic factors and early socialisation. This baseline can only be altered with great difficulty. According to 'set point theory', serious life events may influence an individual's current subjective well-being, but this influence will only be temporary. Thus life events which are viewed positively bring a temporary increase in life satisfaction, while those viewed negatively are accompanied by a drop in the level of life satisfaction.

S. Weick (✉)
Social Indicators Research Centre, Gesis – Leibniz Institute for the Social Sciences,
P.O. Box 12 21 55, 68072 Mannheim, Germany
e-mail: stefan.weick@gesis.org

F. Maggino (ed.), *A New Research Agenda for Improvements in Quality of Life*,
Social Indicators Research Series 57, DOI 10.1007/978-3-319-15904-1_9

In connection with serious illnesses, different empirical findings have been discussed. These suggest that, following the decline in subjective well-being resulting from the need for assistance and care, there is a return to the original baseline. The well-known observation that people with serious spinal injuries do not differ appreciably from the population average (Brickman et al. 1978) in their subjective well-being seems to confirm the hypothesis of a generally valid 'set point theory'. In particular, panel data from Pagán-Rodríguez (2012) and Pagan (2010), showing that people completely adapt to disability about 5 years after the onset, encourages the assumption that – in terms of life satisfaction – people's global satisfaction level recovers even when they need personal assistance or care. Other longitudinal studies partly based on the same base data find no adaptation or only partial adaptation, in terms of satisfaction with life in general, in the years following the onset of disability (Lucas 2007; Oswald and Powdthavee 2008; Powdthavee 2009). The recovery of life satisfactions also depends on personality traits (Boyce and Wood 2011). The different studies do not use the same definitions of disability. The definitions are based on questions about the degree of officially registered disability, work-limiting health conditions and very low levels of health satisfaction. The need for personal assistance or care and thus dependency on others is not taken into account in these studies.

This paper aims to give an overview of the life circumstances of individuals in need of personal assistance, and combines a descriptive section based on a cross-sectional perspective with a section based on panel regression analysis of the change in satisfaction levels. The following research questions are studied:

When does the need for assistance and care arise in the life course?

Which limitations in everyday life can be observed among those affected by the need for assistance and care?

How do people with different degrees of need for assistance and care differ in their satisfaction with life and more specific domain satisfactions?

Do satisfaction with life and domain satisfactions return to their baseline level after the onset of the need for personal assistance and care?

Database

The database for the analyses is the German 'Socio-Economic Panel Study' (GSOEP), the largest longitudinal social science and economic survey of households and individuals in Germany (Wagner et al. 2007). The panel survey allows to determine whether there are people in the households surveyed, in the particular current year, who are permanently in need of assistance and care because of illness, disability or age. Only information from interviewees in private households is taken into account. Household-related data can be analysed in conjunction with the information derived from the personal interviews. Personal questionnaires are used to gather information on the levels of life satisfaction in general, health satisfaction, and satisfaction with other spheres of life. The information on general and domain satisfaction is collected in the personal interview using an 11-step scale from 0 ('completely dissatisfied') to 10 ('very satisfied'). The question about whether any person in a given household is in need of assistance or care is included in the household questionnaire. An additional question addresses the level of assistance needed. The questions were worded differently before 1991. For the analysis of pooled cross-sections, the panel waves of the GSOEP beginning in 1991 are drawn on. Special questions on health limitations were asked in selected years only (2002, 2004, 2006, 2008 and 2010).

For the longitudinal panel regression analysis of changes in life satisfaction, the whole available period of observation in the GSOEP from 1984 to 2011 is used. During this time period, information about levels of life satisfaction from 46,129 interviewees is available for use in the evaluation (379,318 person-years). During this time, 1,817 interviewees (with an examination period of 19,444 person-years) needed assistance or care[1] in at least 2 consecutive years. For the panel regression analysis on adaptation, the event is defined as being in need of assistance or care for at least 2 consecutive years. Single-year periods are dropped from the dataset for the analysis of adaptation. Episodes are only taken into account if the event has occurred for the first time during the observation period. Left-censored cases, where a respondent is already in need of personal assistance when first interviewed in the GSOEP, are also omitted.

Distribution of the Need for Personal Assistance and Care Over the Life Course

This section investigates how widespread the need for personal assistance and care is, and at what age people are affected. The first step is to address the question of prevalence using a cross-sectional perspective. Thus distributions for the year 2011, along with the pooled data from 21 panel waves (1991–2011), are shown in Table 9.1. The pooling is carried out to obtain more stable results with respect to fluctuations between single years, and to achieve higher cell counts. If we investigate how widespread the permanent need for assistance and care because of age, illness or disability is in Germany, we find on the basis of the pooled dataset that 2 % of the population 17 years of age or older is in need of assistance or care. Differences exist with respect to the severity of the impairment and hence also the nature of the assistance required by those affected. Fourteen per cent of the people

[1] The data used in this paper was extracted using the Add-On package PanelWhiz for Stata. PanelWhiz (http://www.PanelWhiz.eu) was written by Dr. John Haisken-DeNew (john@PanelWhiz.eu). See Haisken-DeNew and Hahn (2006) for details. The SOEPMENU-generated Do file to retrieve the SOEP data used here is available from the authors upon request. Any data or computational errors in this paper are our own.

Table 9.1 Need of personal assistance and care in private households

	2011 (%)	1991–2011 (%)
Percentage of people needing assistance and care:		
The interviewee is in need of assistance/care	1.7	2.0
Other person in household	2.0	2.2
Need of assistance/care:		
Shopping outside the home	10	14
Housekeeping/meals	17	27
Basic care (help with getting dressed/undressed; washing oneself)	47	36
Serious care (being moved from one bed to another)	26	23
Number of observations	25,335 (408)	468,310 (7,135)
Number of persons	25,335 (408)	58,285 (2,284)

Database: German Socio-Economic Panel Study (GSOEP) 2011 and pooled cross sections 1991–2011

who require assistance only need help with shopping and errands outside the home; 27 % require support in their housekeeping and in the provision of meals and drinks. The largest group (36 %) needs basic nursing care, for example help with personal hygiene and with dressing and undressing. Twenty-three percent of all those in need of assistance require nursing services, which include comprehensive daily care and other services such as being moved to another bed.

When does the need for personal assistance and care occur over the life course? The next step is to address his question by means of event history analysis. The first time a person observed in the GSOEP needs personal assistance and care for two consecutive years is defined as the event, and the age of the respondent is defined as the analysis time. The survival curve estimate (Graph 9.1) demonstrates the rapid increase in the proportion of persons affected after the age of 80 years. The fact that this occurs primarily in old and very old age constitutes a major difference between this group and the disabled individuals examined in existing studies on persons of working age.

Another important question is related to the transitions between the different degrees of need for personal assistance and care. How likely is it that the situation will improve or worsen? Table 9.2 shows the transition probabilities of each outcome (1984–2011). The diagonal of the values of the table in bold letters indicates the probability of staying on the same level, which is more than 50 % on the two highest levels. For the lower levels the likelihood of a transition to a greater degree of need for personal assistance is higher than the likelihood that the situation will improve. The probability of moving directly out of the need for personal assistance is very low for those in the two highest grades, but the probability of an improvement (to a lower degree of need for assistance – Table 9.2 last row: 2.6 + 1.2 + 3.4 + 15.8) is as high as 23 % for those needing a high level of nursing care.[2]

[2] The higher the degree of need for personal assistance, the higher the probability of non-response in the subsequent panel waves.

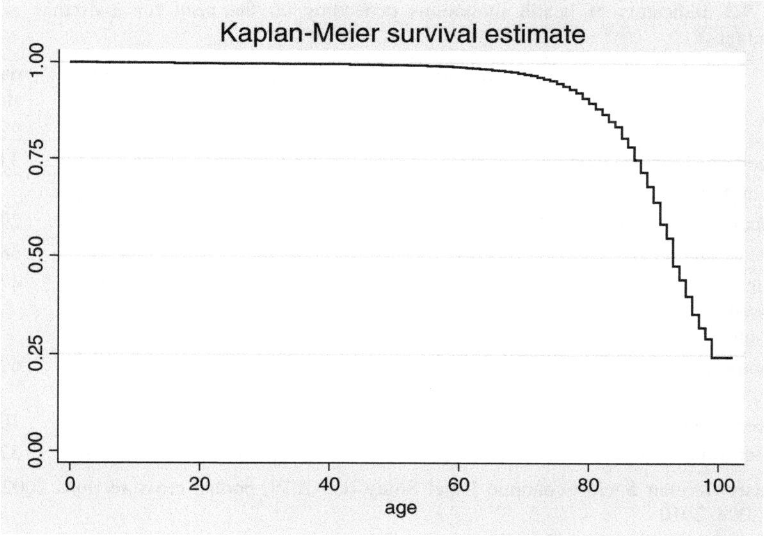

Graph 9.1 First occurrence of need of personal assistance and care over the life course (Database: German Socio Economic Panel (GSOEP) 1984–2011 (own calculations))

Table 9.2 Transition probabilities between different grades of the need of personal assistance and care in %

Need of assistance/care:	0	1	2	3	4	No observation
0 – No need of assistance/care	**91.8**	0.1	0.1	0.1	0.0	8.0
1 – Shopping outside the home	15.5	**31.2**	23.8	13.7	3.8	11.9
2 – Housekeeping/preparing meals	8.8	8.7	**44.0**	17.3	8.2	13.1
3 – Basic care (help getting dressed/ undressed, washing oneself)	4.3	2.5	10.2	**52.7**	14.5	15.8
4 – Serious care (being moved from one bed to another)	2.6	1.2	3.4	15.8	**53.3**	23.7

Database: German Socio-Economic Panel Study (GSOEP) 1984–2011
Number of observations: 420,627; number of persons: 47,810

Health Limitations of People in Need of Personal Assistance and Care

The Socio-Economic Panel Study also offers, at least cross-sectionally, several indicators of health limitations which help to describe the situation of persons in need for assistance or care more precisely. Crucial in this context is the limitation of

Table 9.3 Indicators of health limitations depending on the need for assistance and care (percentages)

	Impairment of the ability to climb stairs	physical pain in the last 4 weeks	Limited social contacts	poor state of health
No need of assistance/care	10.6	13.7	6.4	3.6
Need of assistance/care:				
Shopping outside the home	71.4	48.1	30.7	29.8
Housekeeping/meals	76.1	49.0	44.3	38.8
Basic care (help with getting dressed/undressed; washing oneself)	87.4	53.6	52.0	47.8
Serious care (being moved from one bed to another)	87.9	62.3	66.4	67.4
Number of observations	106,586	106,213	106,243	106,671
Number of persons	32,780	32,756	32,746	32,788

Database: German Socio-Economic Panel Study (GSOEP), pooled cross sections 2002, 2004, 2006, 2008, 2010

mobility as it is a major reason why people need assistance from others. Roughly 80 % of those needing care due to age or sickness complain of increased impairment of their ability to climb stairs. Alongside mobility limitations, the daily routines of people who are dependent on support are also marked by pain: about half of those polled had suffered physical pain, either constantly or at least often, in the 4 weeks preceding the survey. Three quarters of those individuals who are dependent on serious nursing care services are especially affected by this. Not surprisingly, this has additional effects on all aspects of their lives, including their participation in social life. With the growing need for assistance and care due to age or sickness, social contacts become increasingly rare. Of those individuals who require serious nursing care services, three quarters had always or at least often experienced limitations in their social contacts in the last 4 weeks. Despite the considerable limitations experienced by those in the less severe category, those affected do not for the most part judge their state of health as poor. Only those individuals who require serious nursing care judge their state of health as mainly poor. It is very likely possible deteriorations in one's own state of health are taken into consideration (Table 9.3).

Satisfaction Levels at Different Degrees of Need for Personal Assistance and Care

In a group-specific view of pooled cross sections, the need for personal assistance and care goes hand in hand with low levels of subjective well-being. General life satisfaction decreases in proportion to an increased need for personal assistance and care. For people who require support in the form of serious nursing care, the average is 4.3, more than two and a half points below the average level of

Table 9.4 Average satisfaction according to need of assistance/care 1991–2011

	Satisfaction with life in general[a] (0–10)	Satisfaction with life expected in 5 years[a] (0–10)	Satisfaction with health[a] (0–10)	Satisfaction with household income[a] (0–10)
Need of assistance/care:				
No need of assistance/care	7.0	6.9	6.6	6.2
Shopping outside the home	5.5	4.9	3.3	5.9
Housekeeping/preparing meals	5.3	4.8	3.2	6.0
Basic care (help with getting dressed/undressed; washing oneself)	5.1	4.3	2.9	5.9
Serious care (being moved from one bed to another)	4.3	3.8	2.1	5.9
Number of observations	379,400	290,836	379,649	373,501
Number of persons	48,686	46,876	48,709	48,321

Database: German Socio-Economic Panel Study (GSOEP) pooled dataset 1991–2011
[a]Scale from 0 "completely dissatisfied" to 10 "completely satisfied"

satisfaction experienced by people who have no need of assistance (Table 9.4).[3] The difference in life satisfaction between those with the highest and lowest degrees of need of care dependency is 1.2 scale points on the 11-point scale, which indicates additional significant differences in people's subjective well-being. Subjective well-being in difficult situations depends not least upon how people judge the likely subsequent development of their living situation. What expectations for the future do people in need of personal assistance and care have? A look at the life satisfaction expected in 5 years shows a subdued, pessimistic view – it is about half a point below the current level of life satisfaction. Thus respondents seem quite aware that can be their living conditions are likely to deteriorate. As expected, respondents' assessments of their health turn out to be especially unfavourable. The specific level of satisfaction with their own health, at points far below the midscale, is clearly below the level of life satisfaction, though the range within the varying degrees of need for personal assistance is no greater than that within varying levels of life satisfaction. The position relative to interviewees who have no need of assistance is, however, extremely pronounced. The difference between those without care needs and those with the highest needs is 4.5 points. The equivalent difference in terms of life satisfaction is 2.7 points. One can imagine that a low quality of life for persons in need of assistance and care is not always sudden and might be preceded by a more or less continuous deterioration of their health situation, resulting in decreases in subjective well-being as well as possible adaptations over time. This is not taken into account in a cross-sectional group comparison.

[3] Significance level of all reported differences: $p < 0.001$.

Changes in Life Satisfaction After the Onset of the Need for Personal Assistance and Care

The longitudinal perspective is of major relevance. This is partly because of the inaccurate picture that may be given by one or more cross-sectional snapshots, encouraging a tendency to overestimate long-term cases and to hide developments. It is also relevant from a theoretical perspective, when assumptions are being made about how subjective well-being, having fallen with the onset of the need for assistance or care, may recover again. The theoretical models explaining subjective well-being are based on assumptions about reactions and adaptations over time. The next step will be to examine how people's general level of life satisfaction changes over time when the event need for personal assistance and care occurs, that is, when time sequences are taken into consideration. According to set point theory, deviations from the baseline are temporary – i.e., even following decisive life events, people adapt to their objective circumstances, after which their life satisfaction returns to its original level. With the GSOEP data used here we can access a long observation period that allows us to take into account changes affecting people who initially require no assistance, and also to study developments following the onset of the need for assistance and care.

In the following section, regression models for panel data with fixed effects for individuals will be used to examine the average change in levels of satisfaction with life, health and household income in comparison with the baseline for varying degrees of need for assistance. The selection of independent variables follows Pagán-Rodríguez (2012), with the difference being that leads and lags are estimated in the same equation here. The analysis is restricted to the first episode of need for assistance and care occurring during the observation in the panel study, and to non-left-censored cases. All persons at risk of needing personal assistance or care are included in the analysis.[4] Besides general life satisfaction (model 1), satisfaction with two specific life domains, health (model 2) and household income (model 3), are analysed by separate regressions. The inclusion of the models with the two domain satisfactions is supposed to give a more detailed view of how these different aspects of subjective well-being are related to the more general evaluation indicated by satisfaction with life in general.

The regression parameters for the current need for assistance show the deviation in the level of life satisfaction from the baseline. In addition, a possible change in the level of life satisfaction in the years before the onset of need is also examined by means of four dummy variables (leads). An adaptation to the deterioration in one's living situation is recorded using dummies for the duration of the need for assistance (lags). Additional influence factors for life satisfaction have been controlled for (Table 9.5). 'Set point theory' is based on a long-term individual baseline of

[4] Weick (2012) analysed life satisfaction after the onset of the need for personal assistance and care on the basis of the waves of the GSOEP from 1992 to 2004, and also found a substantial decrease in life satisfaction with no linear effect of adaptation over time. The lead effect was controlled for 1 year. The analysis was not restricted to the first episode of the need for personal assistance and care, and the independent variables used were different.

Table 9.5 Panel regression analyses of changes in life satisfaction occurring with the incidence of the need for assistance/care

	Model 1	Model 2	Model 3
	Satisfaction with life in general	Satisfaction with health	Satisfaction with household income
Current need of assistance/ care:	−0.83***	−1.37***	−0.10
Shopping outside the home			
Housekeeping/meals	−1.36***	−1.74***	−0.07
Basic care	−1.72***	−1.98***	−0.10
Serious care	−2.56***	−2.57***	−0.31**
Leads			
Disabled 4 years hence	−0.12*	−0.26***	0.05
Disabled 3 years hence	−0.40***	−0.54***	−0.04
Disabled 2 years hence	−0.36***	−0.66***	0.00
Disabled 1 years hence	−0.90***	−1.23***	0.00
Lags			
Disabled 1 years	−0.00	−0.12	−0.06
Disabled 2 years	0.07	0.21*	−0.02
Disabled 3 years	0.17	0.25*	−0.07
Disabled 4+ years	0.18*	0.41***	0.01
Age			
21–34	0.19***	0.17***	0.39***
35–44	0.14***	0.12***	0.30***
Single	−0.15***	−0.05*	−0.24***
Widowed	−0.17***	0.05	0.19***
Divorced	−0.04*	0.01	−0.37***
Separated	−0.43***	0.01	−0.49***
Years of education	0.01	0.01*	0.03***
Log (real household income per capita)	0.27***	0.09***	0.88***
Number of children			
1	0.02	0.03	0.02
2	0.02	−0.07	−0.10
3+	−0.01	−0.86	−0.74
Household size			
2	−0.01	−0.09***	−0.23***
3	−0.15***	−0.13***	−0.50***
4 + −	−0.22***	−0.16***	−0.57***
Employment status			
Part-time	−0.02	−0.01	−0.05***
Not working	−0.14***	−0.02*	−0.32***
Homeowner	0.07***	0.04**	0.03*
Constant	5.04***	6.68***	−2.71***
Number of observations	377,635	377,818	375,035

(continued)

Table 9.5 (continued)

	Model 1	Model 2	Model 3
	Satisfaction with life in general	Satisfaction with health	Satisfaction with household income
Number of persons	45,877.00	45,898.00	45,750.00
R^2 within	0.04	0.05	0.04

Database: German Socio Economic Panel (GSOEP) 1984–2011 (own calculations)
Fixed effects panel regression, year dummies and dummy for East-Germany included in equations
$^{*}p < 0.05$, $^{**}p < 0.01$, $^{***}p < 0.001$

satisfaction from which temporary deviations may be expected during significant life events. Adaptation or partial adaptation would be indicated by a significant positive effect of the duration dummies.

The coefficients in Table 9.5 show the deviation from the baseline in the metric of the satisfaction scale. Model 1 shows a significant decline in life satisfaction during periods marked by the need for assistance and care. The greater the current need for assistance, the greater the deviation from the baseline. Even at the lowest degree, where support with shopping and errands outside the home is required, the individual level of life satisfaction drops down to 0.83 points below the baseline. At the highest degree of assistance needed, that of *serious* nursing care, which includes, for example, help with moving from one bed to another, the level of life satisfaction drops as far as 2.56 points below the baseline. The need for assistance and care thus goes hand in hand with marked losses in life satisfaction. There is also a distinct anticipation effect before the onset, with life satisfaction declining by 0.9 points 1 year before the need for assistance arises. This justifies the conclusion that an individual's situation is already deteriorating before the onset of need. In fact a decline in life satisfaction can be observed up to 4 years before the onset.

One central question addresses adaptation to the changed living conditions that accompany serious illness and dependence on the help of other people. A rebound in life satisfaction in the case of those in need of assistance or care over the course of several consecutive years could not be observed. The effects of the dummy variables for the lags indicating the duration of the individual's need for assistance fail to become significant, except the one for being disabled for 4 years or more. Despite the long time span, which gives subjects the chance to adapt to the objective situation, the effect is small (+0.18). Compared to the strong effects of being in need of assistance (−2.56 for serious care), this is only a minor improvement. The lack of adaptation to this particular situation involving illness and disability also represents an important precondition for the striking group-specific differences in the cross-section between people who need assistance and those who do not.

In model 2, health satisfaction is defined as the dependent variable. As in model 1, health satisfaction decreases with the level of the need for assistance, although among the lower levels of the need for assistance, the negative effects are stronger than in the case of life satisfaction. The occurrence of the need for assistance with shopping outside the home comes with a decline in life satisfaction of 0.83 on the 11-point scale, while the decline in health satisfaction is 1.37. For persons in need of serious nursing care, however, the effects do not differ between health and life satisfaction. This can be interpreted to mean that the different domains of life are affected so seriously that the overall life evaluation is affected as much as the specific health evaluation. The stronger lead effects in model 2 contribute to the assumption that an already worsening health situation in the years before the onset of the need for personal assistance is perceived particularly negatively in the health evaluation and to a lower degree in the overall life satisfaction. Interestingly, though, the lag effects in model 2 are also greater than in model 1. This indicates more adaptation in health satisfaction than in life satisfaction, but it is still far from full adaptation. After 4 years (or more), health satisfaction recovers only about 0.4 points, which means that health satisfaction remains more than two scale points lower than the baseline (Graph 9.2).

Income satisfaction is much less affected by the onset of the need for assistance and care, as this does not lead to a decline in household income. Persons affected are usually far beyond retirement age and do not have to face a transition out of employment accompanied by a drop in income. On the other hand, dependency on others might mean higher consumption expenditures, as nursing services or other assistance from the market are unlikely to be fully compensated by nursing care allowances. But it seems that all the other facets of the situation of needing assistance and care overshadow the economic domain. Only in the case of serious care is the relevant effect significant (−0.31) and much smaller than in model 1 or model 2. No evidence can be found for anticipation or adaptation. Lead and lag effects are not significant in model 3. In the context of the major problems in everyday life which come with the onset of the need for personal assistance and care, the economic domain seems to play a minor role in people's evaluation of their lives.

Conclusions

Being in need of personal assistance and care can be characterised by a constant decline in subjective well-being which seems to be different to the situation of working age males who become disabled but adapt fully with respect to life satisfaction after 5 years as the study of Pagán-Rodríguez (2012) shows. This might have to do with the definition of disability used, but it mainly reflects the fact that the disabled in the study of Rodriguez are younger and more resilient than those in need of personal assistance and care. Moreover, transitions of the disabled out of employment going along with fewer responsibilities might make it easier to meet everyday requirements and thus encourage adaptation processes.

Following Veenhoven (2005), the distinction between needs and wants is of some importance. Germany as an affluent welfare state ensures that basic needs are met even if officially registered disabled are in such poor health that they are no longer able to be gainfully employed. Beyond this level of needs gratification, adaptation can be observed. On the other hand, the impairments of those in need of

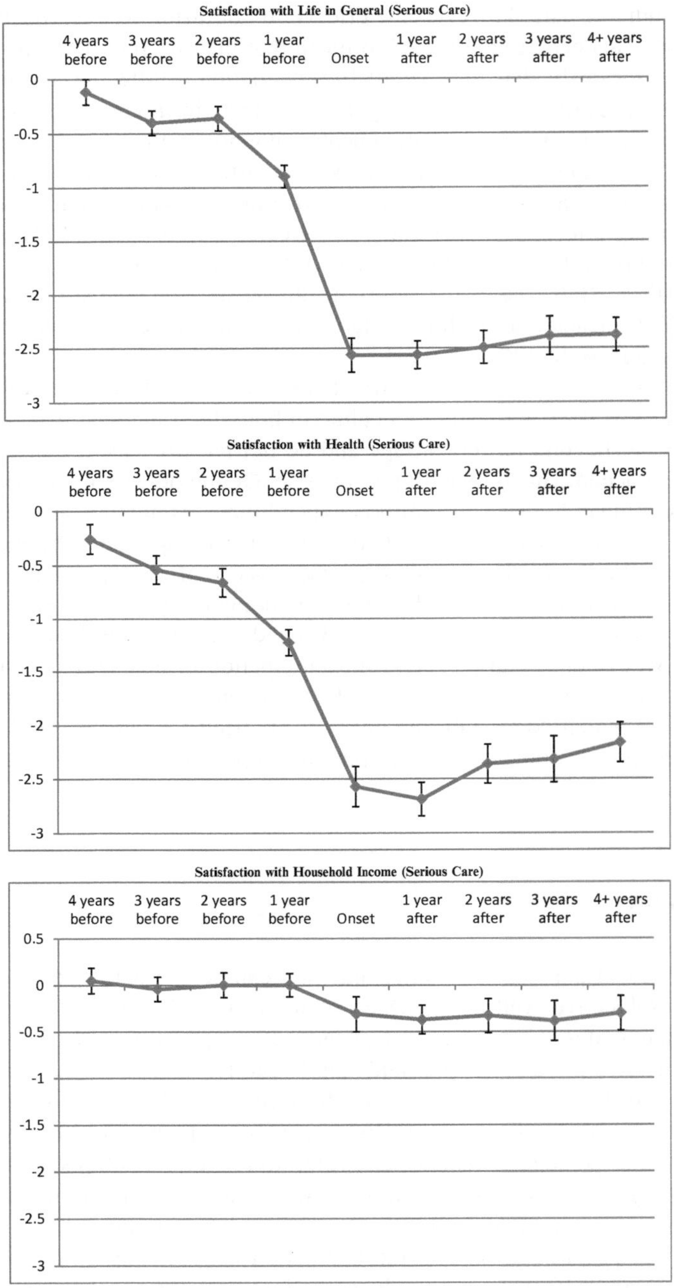

Graph 9.2 Dynamic effect of the onset of the need of personal assistance and care (Database: German Socio Economic Panel (GSOEP) 1984–2011)

personal assistance and care due to sickness and old age are obviously so serious that their aspiration levels cannot be adapted to this life situation, because their basic human needs are not being met. Easterlin (2003) stresses the fact that aspiration level adaptations particularly emerge when material living conditions are involved but to a far lesser extent in the family or health spheres. It has been shown that persons in need of personal assistance and care are severely restricted in their mobility, suffer physical pain and only have limited social contacts. Even in late life the inner psychological mechanism for sustaining an individual level of satisfaction obviously does not take hold here. In such a situation, life satisfaction can only be expected to return to a higher level if the objective living conditions improve. The need for assistance or care implies – in varying degrees – dependency on other people in one's daily life, and affects nearly all life domains, while economic aspects seem to be of minor importance. It has been shown, that persons in need of personal assistance and care do not judge their health situation as bad as one might expect. It can be assumed, that this is a result of mechanisms of social comparisons. Persons in need of assistance can realise their adverse living conditions compared to most others, but might be aware of even worse situations of other sick and old persons and take into account a possible deterioration of their own living conditions. With the help of others those observed in this study still live in their usual living environment in private households. Nonetheless these life circumstances have serious effects on subjective well-being. Further research might also address subjective well-being of persons in need of personal assistance and care going along with transitions from private households to residential care.

References

Boyce, C. J., & Wood, A. M. (2011). Personality prior to disability determines adaption: Agreeable individuals recover lost life satisfaction faster and more completely. *Psychological Science, 22*, 1397–1402.

Brickman, P., Coates, D., & Janoff-Bulmann, R. (1978). Lottery winners and accident victims: Is happiness relative? *Journal of Personality and Social Psychology, 36*, 917–927.

Diener, E., Lucas, R., & Scollon, C. (2006). Beyond the hedonic treadmill: Revising the adaptation theory of well-being. *American Psychologist, 61*, 305–314.

Easterlin, R. A. (2003). Building a better theory of well-being. In L. Bruni & P. L. Porta (Eds.), *Economics and happiness: Framing the analysis* (pp. 29–64). New York: Oxford University Press.

Haisken-DeNew, J. P., & Hahn, M. (2006). *PanelWhiz: A flexible modularized Stata interface for accessing large scale panel data sets.* http://www.PanelWhiz.eu

Headey, B. (2006). *Life goals matter to happiness. A revision of set-point theory* (DIW Discussion Paper 639). Berlin: Deutsches Institut für Wirtschaftsforschung (DIW).

Lucas, R. (2007). Long-term disability is associated with lasting changes in subjective well-being: Evidence from two national representative longitudinal studies. *Journal of Personality and Social Psychology, 92*(4), 717–780.

Lucas, R. E., Georgellis, Y., & Clark, A. E. (2003). Reexamining adaptation and the set point model of happiness: Reactions to changes in marital status. *Journal of Personality and Social Psychology, 84*(3), 527–539.

Oswald, A., & Powdthavee, N. (2008). Does happiness adapt? A longitudinal study of disability with implications for economists and judges. *Journal of Public Economics, 92*, 1061–1077.
Pagán-Rodríguez, R. (2012). Longitudinal analysis of the domains of satisfaction before and after disability: Evidence from the German socio-economic panel. *Social Indicators Research, 108*, 365–385.
Pagan, R. (2010). Onset of disability and life satisfaction: Evidence from the German socio-economic panel. *European Journal of Health Economics, 11*, 471–485.
Powdthavee, N. (2009). What happens to people before and after disability? Focusing effects, lead effects, and adaptation in different areas of life. *Social Science and Medicine, 69*, 1834–1844.
Veenhoven, R. (2005). Happiness in hardship. In L. P. Bruni & P. L. Porta (Eds.), *Economics and happiness* (pp. 243–266). Oxford: Oxford University Press.
Wagner, G., Frick, J., & Schupp, J. (2007). The German Socio-Economic Panel Study (SOEP) – Scope, evolution and enhancements. *Schmollers Jahrbuch: Journal of Applied Social Science Studies, 127*(1), 139–169.
Weick, S. (2012). The incidence of the need for personal assistance and care: Objective living conditions and subjective assessments. In S. Salzborn, E. Davidov, & J. Reinecke (Eds.), *Methods, theories, and empirical applications in the social sciences* (Festschrift für Peter Schmidt, pp. 335–342). Wiesbaden: Springer VS.

Chapter 10
Towards Satellite Accounts on Education and Human Capital in OECD Countries

Fabiola Riccardini

Introduction

This work has been carried out, during 2011 and 2012, within the framework of co-operation in the measurement of well-being between ISTAT and OECD and it is part of the work undertaken by OECD Statistical Directorate in the context of measurement work on human capital and followed one of the recommendations of the Stiglitz-Sen-Fitoussi Report, which suggested constructing comprehensive accounts of all the assets of a country in order to assess the sustainability of its development path (Stiglitz et al. 2009).

It reviews some of the national experiences undertaken to construct satellite accounts for education and human capital, in order to put forward possible development of satellite accounts. Such accounts, if implemented in a consistent way, would represent a natural complement the monetary estimates of the stock on human capital presented by OECD (Liu 2011).

Modern human capital theory has a long tradition. Schultz (1961), Becker (1964) and Mincer (1974) first introduced the idea that human capital should be seen as an important driver of economic growth, a notion that has been later developed by several other authors (Roomer 1986, 1989; Lucas 1988; World Bank 2006). Investment in human capital takes various forms: people may attend school, undertake further education, obtain skills at work, or move to jobs that offer greater opportunities for training. All these activities increase workers' productive capacity and their earning potential in the future.

The OECD defined human capital as "the knowledge, skills, competences and embodied in individuals that facilitate the creation of personal, social and economic well-being" (OECD 2001). This definition includes a broad range of attributes of

F. Riccardini (✉)
Italian Statistical Institute, ISTAT, Rome, IT, Italy
e-mail: fabiola.riccardini@istat.it

F. Maggino (ed.), *A New Research Agenda for Improvements in Quality of Life*,
Social Indicators Research Series 57, DOI 10.1007/978-3-319-15904-1_10

individuals (such as skills gained through formal education and outside school, as well as people's health conditions) and a broad range of benefits stemming from it.

Measures on human capital may serve many purposes. One is to better understand the drivers of economic growth. Another is to assess the sustainability of a country development path/sustainability, in its intergenerational perspective, is usually understood as requiring that the total stock of resources (or 'capital') available in a country is kept unchanged (on a per capita basis) over time (UNECE, OECD, Eurostat 2009); such assessment requires a measure of the stock of human capital that could be compared to those for other types, a requirement that calls for monetary measures. The capital approach is coherent with the classical development theory strongly focused on investment and capital. Sustainability from the point of view of the capital approach aims at accounting for a broad set of capital assets than those already recognised in the current System of National Accounts. More specifically, a set of environment or natural assets, human capital, social capital should be added to the traditional set of capital assets (financial and economic).

Education is the most important factor shaping human capital and, although the broad OECD definition given above recognises the importance of other elements, the focus in this paper is on education. The importance of education for building those skills and competences that underpin economic production has been investigated for many years. According to Krueger (1999), returns to past investment in education and work experience may account for more than two thirds of a country's national income. Much of the research on human capital has focused on the relationship between formal education and wages, and on people's incentives to invest in education, in particular at the post-secondary level (Boarini and Strauss 2009; Boarini et al. 2009).

Education, however, matters for well-being also beyond its effects on people's earnings and productivity. Education is strongly associated with people's evaluation of life, even after controlling for the higher income associated to better education. More educated people also typically have better health status, lower unemployment, more social connections, and greater engagement in civic and political life (OECD 2010c, 2011b). While the available evidence does not always allow conclusion about the direction of causation between education and these dimensions of quality of life, there is a consensus that education brings a range of returns, monetary and non–monetary, that benefit both the person investing in the education and the community in which they live (Stiglitz et al. 2009).

The OECD has a long tradition of statistical work in education, much of it focused on different physical measures of the quantity (OECD *Education at a Glance* 2011a) and quality of human capital *(PISA, IALS, PIAAC)*. Some of these measures refer to inputs (educational expenditures and school resources, school enrolment), while others refer to outputs (completed years of schooling, graduation rates) and other yet to outcomes (standardized test-measures of people's achievements in literacy and numeracy). At the policy level, the *OECD Innovation Strategy* recommends that public policies equip people with the foundations to learn and develop the broad range of skills needed for innovation in all of its forms, as well as with the flexibility to upgrade these skills to changing market conditions.

The concept of 'human capital' is also at the heart of the notion of intangible assets. Education and training policies, especially in universities and vocational training institutions, provide the basis for developing intangible assets in the innovative business (OECD 2010a, b; O'Mahony 2011). Similarly, *the OECD Skill Strategy* calls for policies to improve the responsiveness, quality and efficiency of learning provision, the transferability of skills, the possibility of accessing learning institutions and the lowering of costs of re-entry. Relevant skills range from basic skills to digital-age literacy, academic skills, technical skills, generic skills, "soft" skills, leadership, managerial and entrepreneurial skills. While measures of some of these skills are available from existing international assessment instruments, measures of soft skills, leadership and managerial skills are currently available only at the national level (OECD 2012).

In all OECD countries, governments play a key role in the provision of educational services. The government, however, is not the only provider, and the mix between private and public provision of educational services varies across countries. These services tend to be large: in 2010, OECD countries spent 6.5 % of their GDP on educational institutions at the primary, secondary and tertiary levels, with more than three quarters of the total provided by public institutions. Traditionally, monetary measures of government-provided services are based on the costs of the inputs used to produce them.[1] This procedure is inadequate for productivity analysis since it ignores changes in efficiency with which various inputs are used in production. An output approach (the value of the outputs produced) for measuring the education services production can be called for. When separate measures of inputs and outputs are employed productivity measures could be established by comparing changes in the volume of inputs and changes in the volume of outputs. The OECD, which has a tradition in developing methodologies for measuring the volume and prices of education output within the System of National Accounts (Schreyer 2010), has underscored the importance of moving towards output-based measures of these educational services, and many countries (e.g. Australia, Sweden and Canada) have started to implement output measures of these services that are independent of the costs of inputs. This procedure attempts to capture changes in output quality (Ahlroth et al. 1997; Atkinson 2005; Collesi et al. 2008; Fraumeni et al. 2008; Gu and Wong 2010).

Satellite Accounts (SA) extend the scope of economic accounts without undermining the usefulness of the core accounts. These accounts have been suggested by many institutions and authors (Commission of the European Communities 2009; Landefeld et al. 2010) as one practical way of moving 'beyond GDP', as they allow integrating some of the social and economic aspects of non- and near-market activities, such as the economy's use of natural resources, the impact of investments in research and development, health care and education.

SA for education describe in a coherent framework the relation between the different aspects of the education system, while preserving a link to the core

[1] The costs include teacher's wages and salaries, households expenditures for school fees and educational material, the consumption of fixed capital (the use of school building).

accounts of the System of National Accounts (SNA). However, no common conceptual framework for education satellite accounts currently exists. National practices in this field typically reflect the specific institutional settings of various countries, and may not appropriate for others. This paper presents an attempt to provide a common framework suitable for comparative analysis.

The paper is organized as follows: section "Measuring human capital: First phase" describes briefly measurement for the stock of human capital produced by OECD in the first phase of their project; section "Why satellite accounts and review of satellite accounts across countries" reviews a number of national experiences in developing education satellite accounts and the main lessons; section "Building up a framework for satellite accounts for education and human capital" presents the building blocks framework for satellite accounts on Education and Human Capital (HC); section "Conclusion and future work" concludes by outlining possible treks for future work in this field.

Measuring Human Capital: First Phase

There are different methodologies to measuring human capital. Approaches based on monetary measures and approaches relay on physical measures. Monetary measures includes estimates based on the indirect or residual approach (e.g. World Bank 2011)[2] and direct measures based on information on its components, as the cost-based approach[3] (e.g. Kendrick 1977) and the income-based approach[4] (e.g. Jorgenson and Fraumeni 1992). Moreover, the indicators-based approach relay on physical measures[5] (e.g. OECD Education at a Glance), further divided by quantity measures (e.g. educational attainment, average year of schooling) and quality measures (e.g. test scores, class size, standardized test-measures of people's achievements in literacy and numeracy)

OECD-STD has built a database on monetary estimates of the stock of HC adopting the lifetime income approach. Main results from this database and estimates are:

1. the value of HC(measured by the income-based approach), even restricted to market returns, is substantially larger than the conventional physical capital.

[2] It is part of the Wealth Accounting developed by the World Bank and it measures the total stock of human capital as the difference between the total discounted value of each country's future consumption flows (as proxy of total wealth) and the sum of the tangible components of that wealth.

[3] It measures human capital on the base of all the costs that are incurred when producing it.

[4] It measures human capital by looking at the stream of future earnings that human capital investments generates over the lifetime of a person. It looks at the output side of human capital production.

[5] It measures human capital through various types of educational characteristics of the population.

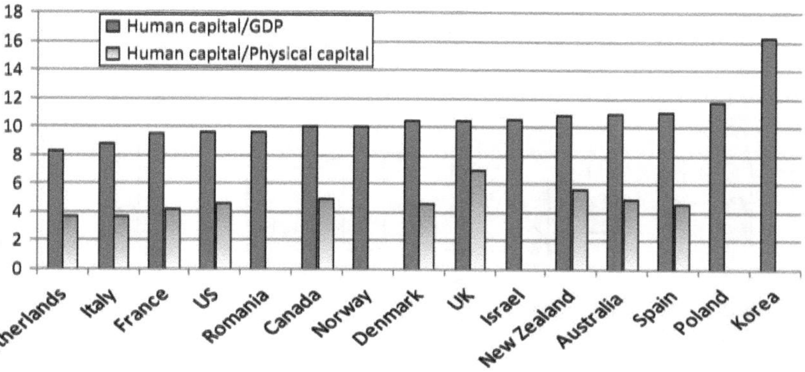

Fig. 10.1 Ratios of human and physical capital to GDP, 2006 (Note: Estimates for Australia refer to 2001, those for Denmark to 2002. Source: OECD, Liu 2011)

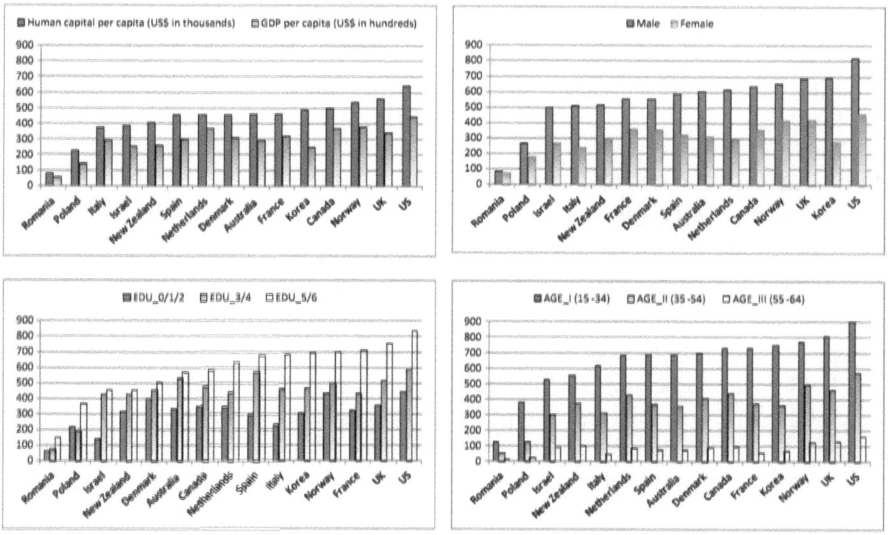

Fig. 10.2 Real human capital per capita (US$ in thousands) in 2006 (Note: Estimates for Australia refer to 2001 and for Denmark to 2002. Source: OECD, Liu 2011)

According to OECD (Liu 2011) the ratio between the stock of human and that of physical capital ranges between 3.6 and 7 %, with a mean of 4.7 % across the countries analysed (Fig. 10.1);

2. the distribution of HC by age, gender and education varies across countries (Fig. 10.2);
3. among the driving forces for change of real HC per capita there are higher levels' of education (influence positively) and ageing population (influence negatively). The magnitude of these forces varies across countries leading to different pattern of HC in different countries (Fig. 10.3).

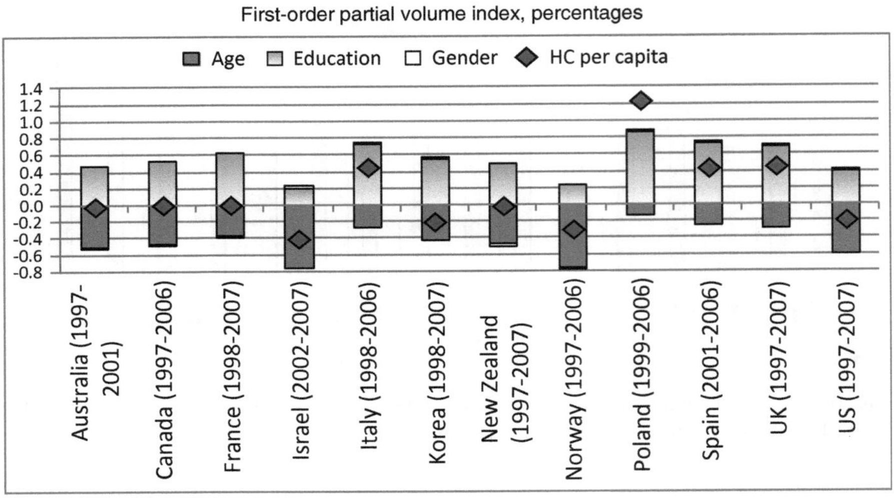

Fig. 10.3 Decomposition of average annual growth of human capital volumes per capita due to age, gender and educational attainment (Note: For many countries, the contribution from gender is to small to e discernable in the figure. Source: OECD, Liu 2011)

Why Satellite Accounts and Review of Satellite Accounts Across Countries

Satellite accounts might allow bringing together in coherent way information on the different aspects connected with the accumulation of human capital, while preserving a link to the core accounts of the SNA 2008.

The flexible framework for constructing of satellite accounts on education and HC, as presented in this paper, represents a pragmatic approach, which consider different levels of definitions and data availability and it is an extension of the OECD Human Capital Project.

In the short-term, this proposal feeds into the CES (Conference of European Statisticians) review on measuring Human Capital. As a matter of fact, the CES suggested to continue on this development (CES 2012).

In the long term this work will contribute to develop measures on sustainability of well-being by enlarging the concept of capital in the SNA (see Box 10.1).

The review of satellite accounts practices involved: France (Ministere Education Nationale Jeunesse 2011), Australia (Wei 2004, 2008), Italy (Di Veroli and Tartamella 2010; Baldassarini and Righi 2011; ISTAT 2011), Netherlands (Bos 2011) and USA (Abraham and Mackie 2005; Abraham 2010; Christian 2011). The analysis of these experiences are reported in the Annex 1, Table A1. The main evidences from those experiences are:

- very few examples of education and human capital satellite accounts have been developed until now, and with different objectives;

- some countries have developed or are in the process of developing basic satellite accounts of education (first type in the terminology of SNA);
- others countries propose to develop more sophisticated models of SA, in which not only market activities are considered, but production and capital boundaries of SNA are changed fundamentally (second type in the terminology of SNA);
- many conceptual and practical difficulties (i.e. methods of estimation, availability of data) are still to be overcome.

The main lesson and possible development from the cases analysed suggest a step by step approach starting from a simple model of SA to arrive to more comprehensive accounting models.

The general objectives of this approach would be:

1. to provide a unified accounting framework, coherent with SNA 2008 for the main monetary and non-monetary aggregates (e.g. the most important factors for human capital formation) and relevant for international and temporal comparisons
2. to provide a flexible tool, expandable by individual countries, for monitoring and analyzing the impact of education services and human capital on economic performance and well-being
3. to provide data for evaluating policies connected to investments in human capital (education policy, fine-tune financing policies in education, labor market, demography, migration, social well-being, growth/sustainability).

Building Up a Framework for Satellite Accounts for Education and Human Capital

In developing a framework for SA is first necessary to consider how Education and Human capital is argued in the SNA 2008. The Box 10.1 summarises some of the key recommendations of SNA 2008 with respect to education, training and human capital.

Box 10.1: The Treatment of Education, Training and Human Capital in SNA 2008

- "It is often proposed that expenditure on staff training and education should be classified as gross fixed capital formation as a form of investment in human capital. The acquisition of knowledge, skills and qualifications increases the productive potential of the individuals concerned and is a source of future economic benefit to them. However, while knowledge, skills and qualifications are clearly assets in a broad sense of the term, they cannot be equated with fixed assets as understood in the SNA, They are acquired through learning, studying and practicing, activities that cannot

(continued)

Box 10.1 (continued)

be undertaken by anyone else on behalf of the student and thus the acquisition of knowledge is not a process of production even though the instruction conveyed by education services is. The education services produced by school, colleagues, universities, etc. are thus treated as being consumed by students in the process of their acquiring knowledge and skills. This type of education is treated as final consumption. When training is given by an employer to enhance the effectiveness of staff, the costs are treated as intermediate consumption" (SNA 2008).

- "This treatment of education costs is consistent with the production and asset boundaries of the SNA but not all uses of the SNA find it satisfactory in all instances. However, as explained below, the SNA in such that users are encouraged to explore alternative conventions in the form al satellite accounts, described in chapter 29. An alternative treatment for the recording of human capital is one such application".
- "An asset is a store of value representing a benefit or series of benefits accruing to the economic owner by holding or using the entity over a period of time..... All assets in the SNA are economic assets (enter in a production process).... The coverage of assets is limited to those assets used in economic activity and that are subject to ownership rights: thus for example human capital as well as natural resources that are not owned are excluded.... it is difficult to envisage "ownership rights" in connection with people, and even if this were sidestepped, the question of valuation is not very tractable."

In the System of National Accounts (SNA 2008), education and training are considered as an element of final consumption expenditure, when undertaken by households, and as intermediate consumption, when the (training) expenditure is incurred by business. Conversely, human capital is not considered as an economic asset because is not subject to ownership rights. The goal of an educational satellite accounts is to go beyond these conventions; this can be achieved by considering education and training as a production process, in which economic units transform inputs in outputs, with the latter representing an investment in human capital. In turn, this implies that human capital should be considered as an asset subject to accumulation, depreciation and revaluation. One implication of this approach, when transferred to the 'core' accounts, is that outlays for education and training (or, at least, part of them) should be considered as capital formation in human capital assets. In an accounting framework, these basic concepts can be developed through a set of satellite accounts with different components.

Definitions and Concepts

Among several definitions in literature the two adopted by OECD are the most meaningful. And give the relevant components of the human capital and the main returns in its investment. In 1998 OECD defined human capital as "the knowledge, skills, competences and other attributes embodied individuals that are relevant to economic activity" (OECD 1998). Later OECD outlined human capital as "the knowledge, skills, competences and attributes embodied in individuals that facilitate the creation of personal, social and economic well-being" (OECD 2001).

Consequently, the **composition** of human capital is related to knowledge, skills, competencies and attributes. In another terms HC includes cognitive skills but also non cognitive skills, such as intra- and inter-personal skills.

Among the **factors** influencing human capital formation and depreciation there are:

- parenting (care from parents for children that influence education and HC formation)
- education (formal education is an investment in HC)
- on-the job training (further improvement of HC derives from the job practice and the training on the job)
- informal learning (other activities beside formal education that increase the knowledge, capacities and abilities of individuals, as for example cultural participation)
- health (better health status imply better learning abilities as well as better job market performances)
- migration (addition to the stock of HC for the country of destination and decrease HC for the country of origin)
- lack of use (decrease HC)
- obsolescence of knowledge (decrease the stock of HC)
- population ageing (decrease the stock of HC)[6]

The **benefits** due to human capital investment can be classified as:

- economic (enhanced employability; allow to earn income and improve career prospects; improve economic situation of people or their productive capacity and contribute to economic production):
  - market (referred to market activities, as...)
  - non-market (referred to non-market activities as household production and free-time)

[6] According to the income-based approach an aged workforce has a shorter expected working period, while younger people have longer periods of lifetime income. But there are other studies that demonstrates countervailing effects, as in A. Righi, M. Montella "Human capital in an ageing society: a multidimensional measurement approach", E-Frame Conference on Measuring Well-being and Fostering the Progress of Societies, Paris June 26–28, 2012.

- non-economic:
  - personal (improve health status, enhance personal well-being)
  - social (better citizens and better parents, greater social inclusion)

However, there is not a clear causal links between each kind of factor influencing HC and the corresponding benefits, mainly because there is still widespread disagreement about the key factors that contribute to human capital formations.

By simplifying we will focus the attention on education as main factor influencing HC formation and economic benefits for individuals as principal return due to HC investment, later enlarging to other factors and benefits taking in consideration data availability too.

In synthesis the basic assumptions are:

1. education is the main factor influencing HC; education is the main driver of human capital investment;
2. distinction between education for final consumption (mostly measured at cost-based approach) and education for investment (mostly valuated at income-based approach);
3. education is looked as a production process, in which economic units transform inputs in output and this output is an investment in HC;
4. human capital is looked as an asset and two definitions are developed: the first one based on the productive capacity embodied in individuals due to knowledge, skills and personal attributes (Schultz 1961; World Bank 2006) and associating the monetary or economic returns (earning capacity, better job), the second one based on the knowledge, skills, competences embodied in individuals that facilitate a broad range of personal, social and economic well-being (OECD 2001) and associating the non-monetary benefits (health, subjective well-being, informed citizens).

All monetary approaches ignore the non-market benefits. This imply to underestimate the value of the stock of HC relative to an ideal concept that would include monetary values of these non-market benefits. Moreover, as we have seen in section "Measuring human capital: First phase", there are different methodologies for developing HC stock value. The monetary measures of the stock of HC have an increased interest because these measures can be compared with those for economic capital based on SNA. The development of satellite accounts is the natural development in this direction and imply an extension of the capital boundaries of economic accounts with respect to HC, as it has been developed in the environmental accounts.

Basic Satellite Accounts

Detailed information on all the financial transactions are the core of this satellite account model and are recorded in the core accounts pertain to the educational sector, distinguishing units by spending, production and financing.

Than transactions are broken down into various levels and subgroups (production units, financing units in terms of institutional sectors) and by sectors and products (e.g. primary education, secondary education, etc.)

Some choices are necessary in the following aspects:

1. Defining boundaries of the educational sector (formal, training) and the various activities connected (teaching, tutoring and secondary activities: canteen, transport);
2. Identifying the units of financing the production of HC (government, non-financial corporations, financial corporations, non-profit institutions serving households and households);
3. Identifying categories of beneficiaries of human capital investment (beyond the standard institutional categories (i.e. resident versus non-resident households, households with different characteristic).

Some examples of "Resources and Use Tables (Tables A.2 and A.3)"[7] and "Supply and Use Table (Table A.4)"[8] are developed in the Annex 1.

In practice, these are satellite accounts in which there is a zooming of the information available in the core of National Accounts, but still education is considered as a final consumption or an expenditure.

More Complex Satellite Accounts

Focusing the attention on monetary returns from investment in HC, a more complex model of satellite account can be developed. In doing this, a basic hypothesis is fixed: all or part of education expenditure should be considered as capital formation in HC. Formal and informal education services has seen as a production process, where people transform inputs into outputs and this output is the investment in HC stock. This asset is subject to depreciation and revaluation (stocks and flows) (Table A.1).

The Production account table should be designed by inputs (market and non-market) and outputs (market and non-market) in the Table 10.1.

Some measurement considerations on the items presented are the following:

1. Market inputs are evaluates on the base of their costs or by the net return to capital and depreciation or at market prices (paid labor of teachers and support

[7] *Resources and use table:* table in matrix form for resources (production) and use (consumption) analysis by products and activities (branches). Each branch can produce, in addition to its distinctive product, also products typical of other branches (along the diagonal you can read the typical productions of each brunch; in the other sections are secondary products, i.e. goods and services produced collaterally to those typical.

[8] *Supply and use table:* represent the flows of goods and services between the supply and the demand side of an economy. They show for a product or a group of products, the amount supplied by producers and the amounts consumed by households, used for investment or exported. They are useful for the analysis of the output (production) and the consumption of goods or services.

Table 10.1 Inputs and outputs of formal education

Inputs	Outputs
Paid labor	Educated individuals
Teachers and support staff	Higher income from being more educated, higher work place and non market productivity
Volunteer labor	Intangibles, better informed citizen, improved individual
Parent time	
Student time	
Materials	
Books and other	
Fixed capital	
School buildings and other structures, equipment, and computer software	
Social capital	

Source: Abraham and Mackie (2005)

staff, materials and fixed capital according to the nature of producer if non-market-public education institution or market-private institution);
2. Non-market inputs are measures by students', parents' and volunteers' time (time spent by people other than students and parents) devoted to education activities multiply for an opportunity cost (i.e. actual wages or future earnings foregone, or a modified opportunity cost) or replacement value (productivity-equivalent replacement wage, that reflect the relative skill of a parent relative to that of the specialist in providing educational services);
3. Output should be estimated by one of the following methods:

- *indicators approach*, total number of students, total number of hours spent by students in each educational activities- with the limit that if class size change and population change there will be a decrease in education output without considering any change in quality – test scores – looking also to the earnings differences with different test scores – in particular is useful to see test score growth rates and valuate with an input expenditure nominal value, taking in consideration quality adjustment;
- *incremental earnings approach*, incremental earnings as a function of additional years of school, or incremental earnings as a function of improvements in test scores;
- *whatever other methods*, that try evaluate returns from investment, or increased productivity of more educated workers. Human capital literature suggests many methods for evaluating the individual returns from investing in education (Abraham and Mackie 2005; Abraham 2010; Christian 2011).

Along with the Production table should be considered the Capital account table by considering depreciation (Graham and Webb 1979; Wei 2008) and revaluation with stocks and flows measures, as in the example of the following sequence (Table 10.2).

Table 10.2 Capital account of human capital

The net value of human capital stock in the opening balance sheet
+ Gross human capital formation in different levels of formal education for the working age population
− Depreciation on human capital formed by education
= Net human capital formation in education
+ Gross human capital formation in on-the-job investment
− Depreciation on human capital formed by on-the-job investment
= Net on-the-job investment
+ Persons turning working age
− Ageing of base level human capital
+ Immigrants
+ Revaluation
Adjusted by
Omissions & errors (including emigrants)
= The net value of human capital at the closing balance

More Advanced Satellite Accounts

Focusing the attention on non-monetary returns from investment in HC, a more complex model of satellite account can be further developed. The two basic table of Production account and Capital account can be modified by:

- Incorporating different factors for human capital formation: education, skills, personality, physical and mental health, social inclusion/capital (OECD 2007, 2010c)
- on the input side should be add rearing costs, health costs for example
- on the output side should be considered that better educated people should show higher level of health and are more likely to exhibit higher level of civic and social engagement

This represent the most experimental side of the satellite accounts, where monetary and non-monetary measures are considered. Nevertheless, many measurement questions are still to be solved.

Measurement Questions

It is obvious that many measurement problems still have to be solved. Here, some of them are listed:

- Many relationships among the various factors that influence human capital should be clarified. Determine the factors of depreciation and revaluation of human capital stock
- Outputs of education might be estimates through the income-based approach or the cost-based approach, therefore it is necessary to explain the differences on these estimates. What are the outputs/outcomes to consider and what methods of estimation (human and social)
- How to estimate non-market inputs, as well as non-market outputs: it is necessary to harmonize methods, for example for non-market production of households
- Understand pricing methods for the different aggregates. What prices/reference values to use? (the question of shadow prices), especially when there are no markets
- How we consider the transnational activities: migration
- Estimation of resource productivity is still controversial
- Discount rate used in stocks estimates is not neutral

Conclusion and Future Work

In this paper has been presented a possible evolution of satellite accounts on Education and Human Capital, for stock and flow measures. This work fits into the measures of sustainability adopting capital approach measures. For the environmental field in 2012 the System of Environmental and Economic Accounts (SEEA) has been agreed, in which natural capital is estimated.

In between of the social and the economic take places the development of satellite accounts on education and human capital. The framework presented here could be a complement to those SA focused on research & development and intangible assets.

The review of the satellite accounts practice has shown that very few example of SA has been developed until now, and with different objectives (France, Australia, Italy, Netherlands and U.S.A.) Many conceptual and practical difficulties (i.e. methods of estimation, availability of data) has to be solved.

Despite the difficulties of measurement and theoretical issues remain unsolved in the paper a basic strategy has been presented for developing satellite accounts on education and human capital based on a gradual strategy, according to specific aims to be pursued, agreement on methods and data availability. This has been presented starting from a simple model of SA to arrive to a more comprehensive accounting model. The general objectives of this approach would be: (1) to provide a unified accounting framework, coherent with SNA 2008 for the main monetary and non-monetary aggregates (e.g. the most important factors for human capital formation) and relevant for international and temporal comparisons; (2) to provide a flexible tool for countries for monitoring and analyzing the impact of education services and human capital on economic performance and well-being; (3) to provide a tool for evaluating policies connected to investments in human capital.

The basic idea developed in the present SA framework try to go beyond the actual accounting of education expenditure or training expenditure in the National Accounts. In particular, education services are considered as a production process, in which economic units transform inputs in output and this output is an investment in HC. Human capital is considered as an asset and two scopes can be developed in SA: the productive capacity embodied in individuals due to knowledge, skills and personal attributes and the knowledge, skills, competences embodied in individuals that facilitate a broad range of personal, social and economic well-being.

In the first model is considered satellite accounts on education zooming information on formal education and this block should be a prerequisite for subsequent blocks. In the second model, is introduced the concept of Human Capital as the productive capacity embodied in individuals due to knowledge, skills and personal attributes and a full set of stock and flow measures are considered, looking to different way to measure input and output of education production, or how to connect stocks and flows related to HC. The third model develops the concept of Human Capital as the knowledge, skills, competences embodied in individuals that enhance well-being in which monetary and non-monetary measures are taken in consideration. Some estimation methodologies are reported and problems connected to each type of SA are pointed out.

In order to implement the above approach, it would be desirable creating a network for sharing experiences and expertise where national accountants, sector experts and scholars would support the development of SA with a building blocks approach. With the support of this network group statisticians should develop guidelines on building SA for education and HC and undertaken experimental estimates in SA for selected OECD countries. These deliverables should reflect and be consistent with policy objectives, existing information, including estimates on non-monetary returns to education.[9]

Developing such databases is important for inter-temporal and international comparisons on education and human capital and for evaluating the impact of investment in education and training on the stock of human capital, on how this investment impacts on the net domestic product and on the net total investment, on what is the productivity in the education sector and its contribution to TFP (Total Factor Productivity), on how human capital can effect on individual, social and economic well-being. The advantage is to have macro measures in the same context which are coherent with the central system of national accounts. Those measures can be useful for researchers, but in particular for policy makers working in a variety of areas, as education (formal and adult training), labour market (for developing skills and job strategies), fiscal policy (to optimise investment in human capital and determine the fiscal impact of government on the private return to education and training), migration and demography policies, and more in general on economic and social well-being. In the knowledge global economy is essential to

[9] This is the way adopted by CES in its November 2012 meeting.

have more clear evidences on people's life deriving from education and human capital investment.

Annex 1: Comparisons from the Analysis of National Experiences on Satellite Accounts in Education and Human Capital and Examples of "Resources and Use Tables" and "Supply and Use Table"

General comments can be deduced from the analyses of national experiences analyzed in Table A.1. Detailed information can be found in the national documentation reported in the references for France: Ministere Education Nationale Jeunesse 2011; for Australia: Wei 2004, 2008; for Italy: Di Veroli and Tartamella 2010; Baldassarini and Righi 2011; ISTAT 2011; for Netherlands: Bos 2011; for USA: Abraham 2005; Abraham 2010; Christian 2011.

Each proposal adds a piece of information for developing SA focused on production, consumption and financing of education services and gradually introducing the concept of human capital. In most of the cases standard production boundary is extended and so is the way assets (human capital) are accounted.

There are different models of SA: some approaches focus only on education, others develop different ways to account for the complex links between education expenditure and human capital see Tables A.2, A.3, and A.4. Some frameworks consider non-market components, while others extend the model by introducing the concept of accumulation and depreciation of human capital.

In general, the level of detail of tables and estimates depends on the aim of the SA, but the availability of data plays an important role too.

Independent estimates of input and output items are needed to evaluate productivity changes in the education sector. An agreement on methodologies (enlarge to non-market components? and how to estimate the single items of production account?) should facilitate this task.

To allow for inter-temporal and country comparisons aggregates should be considered not only at current prices, but also at constant prices.

Table A.1 Comparative analysis of country experiences in developing SA on education and human capital

		Methods			
Country	Objectives of SA	Production/ income/ expenditure	Type of tables	Perspective	Advantages/disadvantages of SA
France	1. Description of financial flows of consumption of education services for analysis of financing and production costs.	Expenditure	1. Financing of educational activities and goods and services	Education	1. Analytical overview for financing and production costs for policies on education
			2. Financing of the sector of production		2. Focused on national education system
			3. Expenditure of sectors of production by activity		
			4. Final and initial financing, transfers between sources of funds		
			5. Educational expenditure in Metropole and in the rest of the world.		
Italy	1. Consider all economic flows of education looking to financing channels and expenditure and classify products, producers, financers	Income/ expenditure	1. Resource/use table by institution producing, 2. by economic activity, 3. supply and use table by product, 4. labour input table	Education versus human capital	1. Analysis for institutional sector and product of financing flows and the main uses of education products
	2. Output of education is an investment in HC evaluated at the production costs				2. Possibility of distinction between market and non market production of educational services
	3. Forecasted a global HC satellite account with connection to non-market production of households and social capital				3. Details on labour inputs for education products
					4. Estimate the value of education production only from an expenditure point of view

(continued)

Table A.1 (continued)

	Objectives of SA	Methods: Production/income/expenditure	Type of tables	Perspective	Advantages/disadvantages of SA
NDL	1. Who pays for HC formation and how education and training are employed in the national economy	Expenditure	1. Supply/use tables	Education + training and Human capital	1. More comprehensive concept of investment in human capital, not only education but also training
	2. Which industry is more HC intensive and allocate HC consumption into various industries or group of persons as a charge on their income		2. Supplementary table on expenditure in human capital		2. Who pay for investment in HC and how education and training are employed in the national economy, through a clear explicitation of labour supply by level of skill too
					3. An attempt to distingue education for final/intermediate consumption and education for productive purpose
					4. Estimate the value of human capital as the sum of expenditures by government, by employers, by households

USA	1. Improve input and output measures by independent methods	Production/ expenditure	Double entry table (national income and production accounts)	Education	1. Independent estimates of input and output and a detailed presentation of different methods for estimate output/ production
	2. Enlarge to non market aspects both for inputs and output of production	Income approach for output			2. There is an attempt to explain why in this type of accounts there is no conceptual identity between returns and cost for investment in education (residual returns or profits of households even if it is controversial)
	3. Education output is the principal factor for investment in HC				3. Suggestion that a full accounting structure will require not only nominal value but also estimates for prices and volume (real value changes over time)
					4. Do not consider the financing flows
Australia	1. Develop an accumulation HC account in which not only formation is considered but also depreciation and revaluation	Income approach for investment in HC	Sort of capital account	Human capital only from post secondary education and working experience	1. Try to integrate stock and flow of HC in a common framework
					2. HC formation derives from population growth and increments to lifetime income

Table A.2 Resources and uses by institution producing education

	Total producers	General Government S13	Central Government S1311 ...	Local Government S1313	Private producers S11 +S15	Non financial corporations S11 ...	NPISHs S15
RESOURCES							
Current transfers/contributions from financing agents (AF)							
AF1							
AF1.1							
...							
Income from sales							
ep1							
ep2							
...							
Capital transfers from financing Agents (donations, non recurrent transfer)							
AF1							
AF1.1							
...							
Other incomes							
USES							
Output of non market sector							
Intermediate consumption							
Consumption of fixed capital							
Taxes on production							
Compensation of employees							
Net operating surplus (market)							

Output of market sector							
Taxes on income etc.							
Current transfer to other sectors and subsectors							
API							
AP1.1							
. . .							
Other expenditures (residual items)							
Gross fixed capital formation							
Balancing item							

Source: Di Veroli and Tartamella (2010)

Table A.3 Resources and uses by main economic activity of producers

	Total producers			General Government producers			Private producers		
	Pre-primary and primary education (NACE rev.1 80.1)	Secondary education (NACE rev.1 80. 2)	Postsecondary and tertiary education (NACE rev1 80 3)	Pre-primary and primary education (NACE rev.1 80.1)	Secondary education (NACE rev.1 80. 2)	Postsecondary and tertiary (NACE rev1 80.3)	Pre-primary and primary education (NACE rev.1 80.1)	Secondary educated (NACE rev.1 80. 2)	Postsecondary and tertiary education (NACE rev1 80.3)
RESOURCES									
Current transfers/ contributions from financing agents									
AF1									
AF1.1									
...									
Income from sales									
ep1									
ep2									
...									
Capital transfers from financing agents									
AF1									
AF1.1									
...									
Other incomes									
USES									
Output of non market sector									
Intermediate consumption									

Consumption of fixed capital									
Taxes on production									
Compensation of employees									
net operating surplus (market activity)									
Output of market sector									
Taxes on income etc.									
Current transfer to other sectors and subsectors									
AP1									
AP1.1									
. . .									
Other expenditures									
Gross fixed capital formation									
Balancing item									

Source: Di Veroli and Tartamella (2010)

Table A.4 Supply and use table for education

	Products			
	ep1	ep2	ep3	ep4
SUPPLY				
Output at basic prices (producers of education)				
API				
AP1.1				
...				
Taxes less subsidies on products				
Imports of education products				
Total supply of education products at purchasers' prices				
USE				
Intermediate consumption				
Final consumption				
Households (S16)				
Government (S13)				
individual				
collective				
Exports of education products				
Capital formation				
Total use of education products at purchasers' prices				

Source: Di Veroli and Tartamella (2010)

References

Abraham, K. G. (2010, April). *Accounting for investments in formal education.* University of Maryland and NBER.

Abraham, K. G., & Mackie, C. (2005). *Beyond the market: Designing nonmarket accounts for the United States.* Washington, DC: The National Academies Press.

Ahlroth, S., Bjorklund, A., & Forslund, A. (1997, March). The output of the Swedish education sector. *Review of Income and Wealth, 43*(1), 89–104

Atkinson, A. B. (2005). *Measurement of government output and productivity for the national accounts* (Atkinson review: Final report). Basingstoke: Palgrave-MacMillan.

Baldassarini, A., & Righi, A. (2011). Verso un conto del capitale umano. In L. Tronti (a cura di), *Capitale umano: definizione e misura.* Milano: Cedam-Kluver.

Becker, G. S. (1964). *Human capital.* New York: Columbia University Press.

Boarini, R., & Strauss, H. (2009). *What is the private return to tertiary education? New evidence from 21 OECD countries.* Paris: OECD Journal, Economic Studies.

Boarini, R., De la Maisonneuve, C., Oliveira Martins, J., & Strauss, H. (2009). *The policy determinants of investment in tertiary education.* Paris: OECD Journal, Economic Studies.

Bos, F. (2011). *A national accounts satellite for human capital and education* (MPRA Eagle Economic & Statistics Working Paper No. 33791). Netherlands.

Christian, M. S. (2011, July). *Human capital accounting in the United States: Context, measurement, and application.* Madison: University of Wisconsin Center for Education Research

Collesi, D., Versace, D., & Zannoni, S. (2008). *Measurement of non-market service: Output and outcomes*. Paper presented for the 30th IARIW conference, Portoroz, Slovenia.
Commission of the European Communities. (2009, August 20). *GDP and beyond – Measuring progress in a changing world*. Brussels, COM(2009) 433 final.
Conference of European Statisticians, Statistical Commission and Economic Commission for Europe. (2012, October 15). Measuring human capital, stock-taking report prepared as a follow-up to the CES 2011 seminar on human capital. ECE/CES/BUR/2012/NOV/11. Geneve
DiVeroli, N., & Tartamella, F. (2010). *The challenge of building education satellite account and the link with human capital account*. IARIW conference, Switzerland.
Fraumeni, B. M., Reinsdorf, M. B.,. Robinson, B. B., & Williams, M. P. (2008, June). *Price and real output measures for the education function of government: Exploratory estimates for primary & secondary education* (NBER Working Paper Series). Cambridge: NBER.
Graham, J. W., & Webb, R. H. (1979). Stocks and depreciation of human capital: New evidences from the present value perspective. *Review of Income and Wealth, 25*(2), 209–224.
Gu, W., & Wong, A. (2010, August 22–28). *Investment in human capital the output of the education sector in Canada*. Paper prepared for the 31st general conference of The International Association for Research in Income and Wealth, St. Gallen, Switzerland.
ISTAT. (2011, June 14–16). Note for Economic Commission for Europe, conference of European Statisticians. *Towards human capital satellite accounting*. Fifty-ninth plenary session, Geneva, Item 5 of the provisional agenda.
Jorgenson, D. W., & Fraumeni, B. M. (1992). The output of education sector. In Z. Griliches (Ed.), *Output measurement in the services sectors*. Chicago: The University of Chicago Press.
Kendric, J. W. (1977). *The formation and stocks of total capital*. New York: Columbia University Press.
Krueger, A. B. (1999). Experimental estimates of education production function. *The Quaterly Journal of Economics, 114*(2), Oxford University Press.
Landefeld, J. S., Moulton, B. R., Platt, J. D., & Villones, S. M. (2010). *GDP and beyond, measuring economic progress and sustainability*. Washington, DC: Bureau of Economic Research.
Liu, G. (2011). *An application of the lifetime income approach to selected countries* (Working Paper No. 41). Paris: OECD.
Lucas, R. E. (1988) On the mechanics of economic development. *Journal of Monetary Economics, 22*, North-Holland.
Mincer, J. A. (1974). *Schooling, experience, and earnings*. Cambridge: National Bureau of Economic Research.
Ministere Education Nationale Jeunesse. (2011). *Le Compte de l'education, Principes, methodes et resultats pour les annees 1999 a 2009*, les dossiers 199 Mai. Paris
O'Mahony, M. (2011). *Human capital formation and continuous training: Evidence for EU countries* (Review of Income and Wealth). Oxford: Blackwell Publishing.
OECD. (1998). *Human capital investment: An international comparison*. Paris: OECD Publishing.
OECD. (2001). *The well-being of nations: The role of human and social capital*. Paris: OECD Publishing.
OECD. (2007). *Understanding the social outcomes of learning*. Paris: Centre for Educational Research and Innovation, OECD.
OECD. (2010a). *The OECD innovation strategy. Getting a head start on tomorrow*. Paris: OECD Publishing.
OECD. (2010b). *Handbook on deriving capital measures of intellectual property products*. Paris: OECD Publishing.
OECD. (2010c). *Improving health and social cohesion through education*. Paris: OECD Publishing.
OECD. (2011a). *Education at glance*. Paris: OECD Publishing.
OECD. (2011b). *How is life?* Paris: OECD Publishing.

OECD. (2012). *Skills strategy, transforming better skills into better economic and social outcomes*. C(2012)48.
Roomer, P. M. (1986). Increasing returns and long run growth. *Journal of Political Economy, 94* (5), 1002–1037.
Roomer, P. M. (1989). *Human capital and growth: Theory and evidence* (Working Paper No. 3173). Cambridge, MA: National Bureau of Economic Research.
Schreyer, P. (2010). *Towards measuring the volume output of education and health services: A handbook* (OECD Statistical Directorate Working Paper No. 31). Paris: OECD.
Schultz, T. W. (1961, March). Investment in human capital. *American Economic Review, 51*, 1–17.
SNA. (2008). *System of National Accounts 2008*. Brussels/Luxembourg/New York/ Paris/Washington, DC: Commission of European Communities-Eurostat/International Monetary Fund/OECD/United Nations.
Stiglitz, J. E., Sen, A., & Fitoussi, J. P. (2009). *Report by the commission on the measurement of economic performance and social progress*. http://www.stiglitz-sen-fitoussi.fr/documents/rapport_anglais.pdf
UNECE/OECD/Eurostat. (2009). *Measuring sustainable development*. New York/Geneva: United Nations.
Wei, H. (2004). *Measuring the stock of human capital for Australia* (Working Paper No. 2004/1). Canberra: Australian Bureau of Statistics.
Wei, H. (2008). *Measuring human capital flows for Australia: A lifetime labor income approach* (Working Paper No. 1351.0.55.023). Canberra: Australian Bureau of Statistics.
World Bank. (2006). *Where is the wealth of nations?* Washington, DC: World Bank.
World Bank. (2011). *The changing wealth of nations: Measuring sustainable development in the new millennium*. Washington, DC: The World Bank.

MIX
Papier aus verantwortungsvollen Quellen
Paper from responsible sources
FSC® C105338
FSC
www.fsc.org

If you have any concerns about our products,
you can contact us on
ProductSafety@springernature.com

In case Publisher is established outside the EU,
the EU authorized representative is:
Springer Nature Customer Service Center GmbH
Europaplatz 3, 69115 Heidelberg, Germany

Printed by Libri Plureos GmbH
in Hamburg, Germany